# DASH DIET FOR TWO

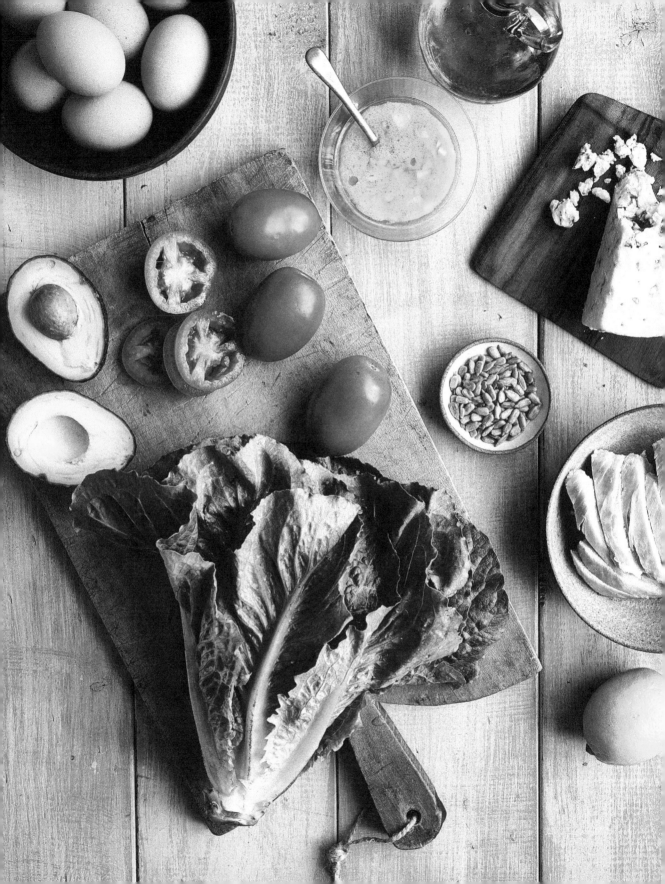

# DASH DIET
## for two

## 125
### Heart-Healthy Recipes to Lower Your Blood Pressure Together

**Rosanne Rust, MS, RDN, LDN**

Photography by Hélène Dujardin

ROCKRIDGE
PRESS

For general information on our other products and services or to obtain technical support, please contact our Customer Care Department within the United States at (866) 744-2665, or outside the United States at (510) 253-0500.

Rockridge Press publishes its books in a variety of electronic and print formats. Some content that appears in print may not be available in electronic books, and vice versa.

TRADEMARKS: Rockridge Press and the Rockridge Press logo are trademarks or registered trademarks of Callisto Media Inc. and/or its affiliates, in the United States and other countries, and may not be used without written permission. All other trademarks are the property of their respective owners. Rockridge Press is not associated with any product or vendor mentioned in this book.

Interior and Cover Designer: Darren Samuel
Art Producer: Meg Baggott
Editor: Anna Pulley
Production Editor: Rachel Taenzler

Photography © 2020 Hélène Dujardin. Food styling by Anna Hampton.
Author photo by Rich Sayer

ISBN: Print 978-1-64739-311-3 | eBook 978-1-64739-312-0

R0

*This book is dedicated to my husband and sons.*
Without their unwavering support, I would not have been able to commit myself as a writer. During the endless hours I spend sitting at my laptop, they pick up the slack. I hope this book makes cooking for two easier for those with high blood pressure and everyone who simply wants to plan healthy meals for two people.

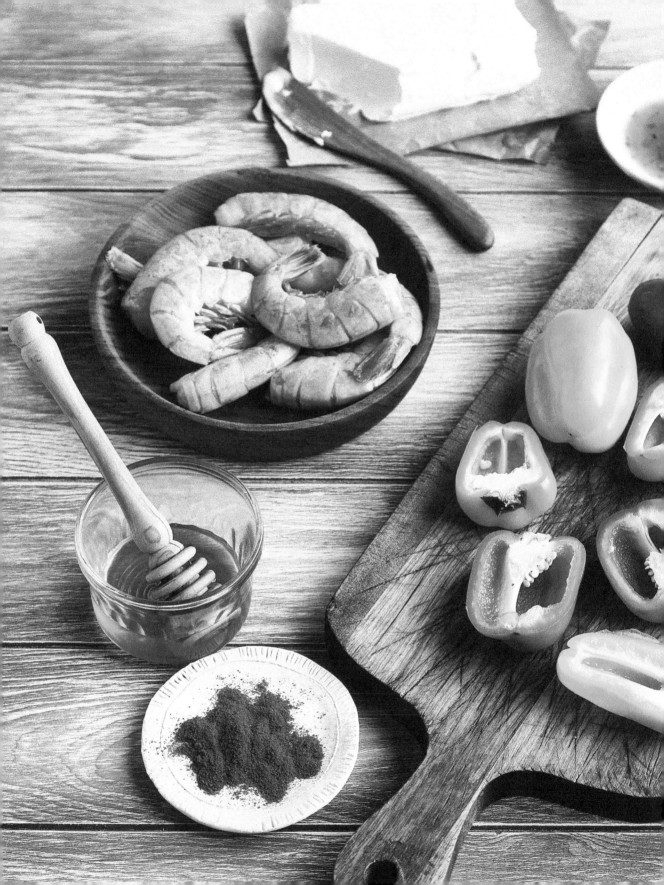

# Contents

# Introduction

Having a strong family history of heart disease, diabetes, and obesity, I was inspired to learn as much as I could about prevention. This was one of the reasons I became a registered dietitian. It's also why I'm so passionate about the DASH diet. As a dietitian, I know that food plays a crucial role in staying well, but sometimes you can't prevent everything. I was diagnosed with high blood pressure after menopause, despite all of my best efforts to eat well, exercise, and prevent it. Oh, the irony! I follow a DASH eating style to keep my blood pressure under control. While I still require medication, following the diet allows me to take a very low dose.

Midlife is a challenging time of transition. I'm sure that at this point in your life you are done spending hours in the kitchen! My goal is to help you enjoy eating well with minimal effort. Whether your children have left the nest, you're planning your retirement, or you've already retired, your health needs should be prioritized now more than ever. Eating well doesn't have to be hard or time-consuming.

Inspired by my Italian roots and trips to Portugal, Greece, and Hungary, this cookbook is designed to help you cook simple and delicious recipes, with practical advice to set you on the path to better health and lower blood pressure. Once you begin a few new habits and incorporate some of my recipes into your weekly rotation, you'll be surprised how easy it becomes. The best part? You'll feel good! You'll also be relieved to know that the road to wellness is not as difficult as you think.

Why the DASH diet? As a science nerd, the fact that DASH has been tested with solid research showing many health benefits—including lowering blood pressure for those with high blood pressure—makes recommending it easy for me. The recipes in this book are specifically designed for two people, making it painless for you to keep your household healthy and stay on budget. This also is a win for the environment, as it helps reduce food waste. When trying to scale down larger recipes to suit two people, you have probably ended up with an accumulation of half-used ingredients in your cabinets. The beauty of recipes for two is that you will not have this issue.

When you make a change in your diet or lifestyle, you need support to be successful. It can be a challenge to shift your culinary style, which is why this book will be a valuable resource. Each recipe is designed to make 2 to 4 servings, with few to no leftovers. Typical cookbook recipes yield 6 to 8 servings, and no one wants to eat the same leftovers for a week, nor waste food. However, some recipes in this book will recommend cooking extra of some ingredients so you can save time and use them in another meal that week. This will give you more leisure time. Who doesn't want more time for fun?

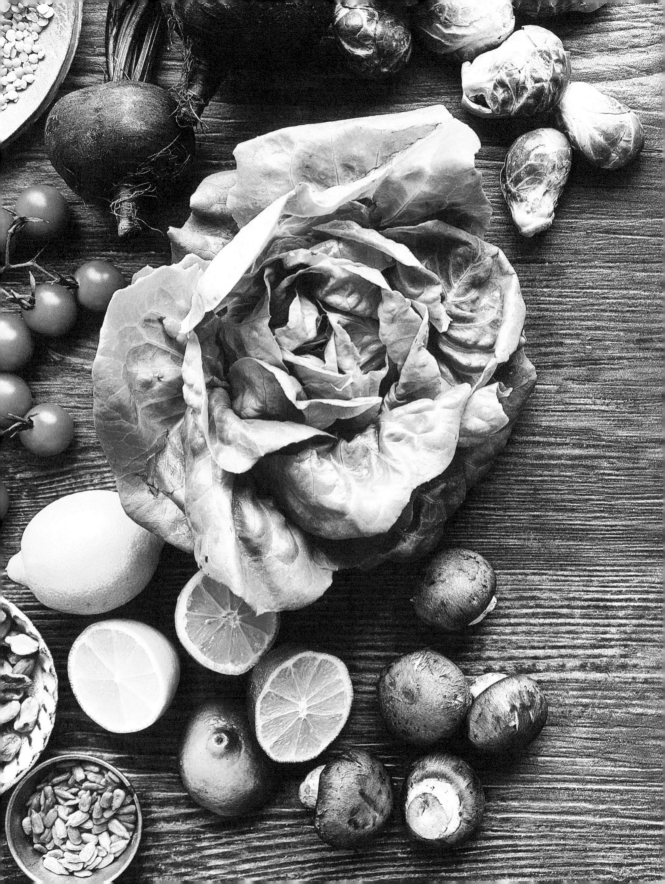

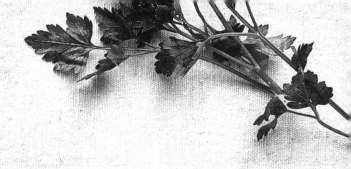

# 1

# THE DASH DIET DEMYSTIFIED

In this chapter, I'll help you understand what the DASH diet is and how it can benefit your health. The DASH eating plan is based on a framework of foods, but it isn't overly restrictive. There'll be no you-absolutely-can-never-eat-that rules in this book. I only suggest that you try to stick to this eating style most of the time (meaning 80 percent or more). You'll be able to enjoy a wide variety of foods on this plan. You may find you eat less of some foods and more of others, but the goal is a balanced plate that lowers blood pressure and keeps you active and healthy.

According to the National Health and Nutrition Examination Survey of 2015–2016, more than 60 percent of all adults over the age of 60 develop high blood pressure. While being overweight increases your risk, you don't have to be overweight to be diagnosed with hypertension. Whether you are approaching midlife, are smack in the middle of it, or beyond, there's a good chance the DASH diet is a good fit for you.

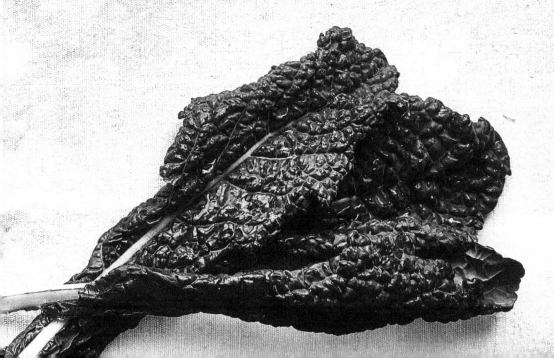

# What Is the DASH Diet?

DASH is not a diet plan based on dashing out the door. It's an acronym that stands for Dietary Approaches to Stop Hypertension. Hypertension is the medical term for high blood pressure. I actually prefer not to call it a "diet," in the sense that the term usually refers to a restrictive weight-loss plan. Instead, think of DASH as a lifestyle choice intended to lower blood pressure and improve your overall health, reducing your risk for heart disease.

The DASH dietary plan is reasonable and balanced, offering you a variety of foods to choose from for any meal or occasion. It emphasizes foods rich in fiber, potassium, magnesium, and calcium. When you think of blood pressure, a low-salt diet may come to mind. Reducing sodium does lower blood pressure in those with high blood pressure, but the DASH eating plan involves much more than just lowering sodium intake. In fact, many people can lower their blood pressure without an extremely low intake of sodium. We'll get to that in a bit.

The eating plan is based on research from a 1997 clinical trial that demonstrated that DASH lowers blood pressure. The study started with feeding a control diet to 459 subjects with high blood pressure for three weeks. The researchers then tested three different diet plans. The control diet was low in fruits, vegetables, and dairy products, and of average fat intake. The study participants were randomly assigned to one of three groups over eight weeks. They either received the control diet again or were in one of two "intervention groups" (either a diet high in fruits and vegetables or a "combination diet" high in both fruits and vegetables as well as low-fat dairy products). Both intervention diets were low in saturated fat.

Among the 133 participants with hypertension (those with blood pressure higher than 140/90 mm Hg), both intervention groups lowered their blood pressure. The diet rich in fruits and vegetables (without dairy) reduced blood pressure, but the combination diet that included dairy reduced systolic and diastolic blood pressure by 11.4 and 5.5 mm Hg more than the control diet. Although participants remained on the DASH diet plan for eight weeks, lower blood pressure was evident in just two weeks. Ongoing research about DASH has confirmed its effectiveness in promoting overall heart health.

If that's not good enough news, there's even better news. A DASH diet plan doesn't just lower blood pressure, it can also help you control your weight, manage your blood sugar, and lower your cholesterol.

## THE STANDARD AMERICAN DIET VS. THE DASH DIET

The Standard American Diet (SAD, no pun intended) differs from a DASH eating plan in a few significant ways. First, most Americans do not eat the recommended servings of fruits and vegetables daily. SAD is also too high in saturated fat and doesn't include enough healthy monounsaturated fats. The common practice of eating processed foods and frequent takeout or restaurant meals means that many people consume high amounts of sodium and way more sugar than is recommended.

These dietary factors (high saturated fat, lack of vitamins, minerals, and fiber, and high sodium and sugar intakes) have the potential to increase the risk of disease in some people. DASH encourages you to include more whole foods (fruits, vegetables, grains, nuts, and seeds), choose healthy fats (monounsaturated fats like vegetable oils, avocados, olives, nuts, and seeds), and reduce portions of meats, sweets, and salty foods.

## DASH HEALTH BENEFITS

An expert panel has ranked DASH in the top two overall diets for several years in a row. *U.S. News & World Report* publishes their review of "best diets" every year, and DASH has been consistently in the number one or two position for almost a decade. Why? It's a sensible, healthy eating plan that's easy for most people to follow. Since it's not overly restrictive, people can stick with it.

Adopting an eating plan based on DASH doesn't just help people lower their blood pressure. Some of the other major benefits include the following:

### Prevent Heart Disease and Strokes

Heart disease and stroke are two of the leading causes of death in the United States. Since high blood pressure is a primary risk factor, modifying your diet and lifestyle can help control this risk. It's worth noting that high blood pressure is also a risk factor for kidney disease, so DASH will reduce your risk for that condition, as well.

While follow-up research about DASH showed it can help lower blood cholesterol and reduce weight (both heart-disease risk factors), other studies showed a positive correlation between the diet and reduced heart-disease risk. The OmniHeart study (Optimal Macronutrient Intake Trial for Heart Health) compared three DASH-inspired diets with different carbohydrate, protein source, and fat parameters. One diet was rich in carbohydrates, one rich in protein (half from plant sources), and one rich in monounsaturated fat. All three diets lowered blood pressure and also lowered Low Density Lipoprotein (LDL), the "bad" cholesterol. (More on this later in this section.)

### Healthy Weight Management

DASH can help you maintain a healthy weight because it's high in fiber and well balanced for all nutrients. Fiber helps keep you full longer, and when you balance your plate at meals with low-fat protein and healthy fats, you won't get hungry as quickly. Also, when you begin to balance your meals, you'll have fewer cravings. As you may know, the calories from sugar and sweets quickly add up. Since sugar is reduced with DASH, the meal plan can potentially result in weight loss.

## Lower Levels of Bad Cholesterol

DASH can control or lower the levels of "bad" cholesterol, a.k.a. LDL cholesterol. A healthy LDL should be less than 100, but you should check with your doctor to determine your overall risk. DASH likely lowers LDL because the plan is low in saturated fat. Fiber also helps lower blood cholesterol levels, so the added whole grains, beans, vegetables, and fruits are all good!

## Lower Risk/Control Type 2 Diabetes

DASH may also help lower the risk of type 2 diabetes. Since the diet is balanced and low in sugar, it's a good choice for anyone with diabetes. Since fruit is higher in sugar than vegetables, it's best to meet your fruit/veggie goals by including more vegetables. Aim for 5 to 6 servings of vegetables and 2 to 3 servings of fruit per day. Check in with a Certified Diabetes Care and Education Specialist (CDCES), however, for your individual dietary needs.

## DASH FOOD GUIDELINES

There are lots of foods that you can eat freely on DASH. The following are the basics to get you started.

## Eat a Variety of Fruits and Vegetables, Including Beans and Legumes

Fruits and vegetables are high in potassium and also provide you with vitamins A and C and other healthy antioxidants. Beans and legumes, which are both high in protein and fiber, also count toward the overall target to increase vegetable intake. Goal: 8 to 10 servings daily.

### Add Low-Fat Dairy to Your Meal Plan

In the DASH research studies, participants experienced lowered blood pressure by increasing their consumption of fruits and vegetables. However, the addition of low-fat dairy products lowered blood pressure even further. I often incorporate Greek yogurt and milk into my recipes, but these foods can serve as snacks, too. If you are lactose-intolerant, look for low-lactose or lactose-free milk brands. If you are vegan or typically use plant-based milk for other reasons, that's fine. However, keep in mind that milk alternatives don't have the same blood pressure–lowering effect or nutrition profile that dairy products do. Goal: 2 to 3 servings daily.

### Reduce Your Portions of Beef, Pork, Poultry, and Fish

Meats such as bacon, sausage, pepperoni, salami, bologna, and other deli meats are higher in saturated fat and sodium, and mostly off-limits. Look for fresh, lean cuts of beef (round, flank, sirloin, tenderloin) and pork (loin, tenderloin) and trim any visible fat. Poultry should also be trimmed of fat and skin. Avoid pre-flavored meats (such as seasoned pork tenderloin or chicken), as these are much higher in sodium. Using your own seasonings will add flavor to these cuts quickly, without the extra sodium. Plus, it will save you money. Fish, especially fatty fish (salmon, mackerel, sardines, anchovies, tuna, trout), is considered to be heart-healthy because of its high omega-3 fatty acid content. Goal: 5 to 8 ounces or less daily.

### Swap Saturated Fats for Unsaturated Fats

Saturated fat is found in foods like butter, coconut oil, lard, margarine, full-fat dairy products, and meats. While it's okay to use small amounts of these foods occasionally, you'll want to stick with nonfat or low-fat dairy and unsaturated vegetable oils (olive oil, canola, or avocado) for the majority of your cooking. A serving is considered to be one teaspoon. Goal: 2 to 3 servings daily.

### Include Nuts and Seeds

Nuts and seeds are another source of monounsaturated fats. They're also high in fiber. You can include nuts occasionally as a snack or use small amounts in your recipes. Goal: 4 to 5 servings a week.

### Focus on Reducing Salty Foods

While the American Heart Association recommends 1,500 milligrams of sodium a day, DASH research suggests that an intake of 3,000 milligrams per day still lowers blood pressure. Reducing your sodium intake will lower blood pressure, but you don't have to completely eliminate salt from your cooking. Pay attention to how much salt you use and look at the sodium content on food labels. For reference, one teaspoon of salt has 2,300 milligrams of sodium. Goal: 1,500 to 3,000 mg of sodium daily.

### Reduce Sugar and Find Alternatives for Sweets

If you have a sweet tooth, have no fear. You can still enjoy some desserts or sweet treats occasionally. I've included a whole chapter of desserts that will inspire you to modify some

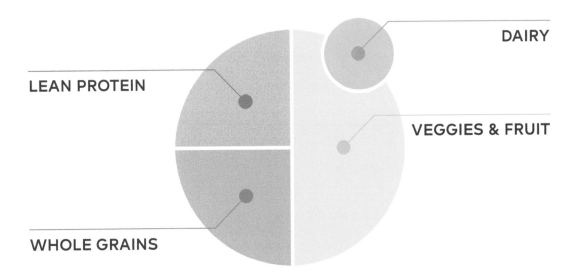

DAIRY

LEAN PROTEIN

VEGGIES & FRUIT

WHOLE GRAINS

of your own favorites. The American Heart Association recommends limiting *added* sugar to 100 calories (six teaspoons of granulated sugar) per day for women and 150 calories (nine teaspoons of granulated sugar) for men. It might be of interest to note that 12 ounces of regular soda contain 150 calories of added sugar. Goal: Limit sugary foods in the diet to twice a week and avoid sugary drinks.

## DASH Cooking for Two

Most cookbooks provide recipes that make 6 to 8 servings. This book is specifically designed to feed two people. As such, the recipes make 2 to 4 servings. For the meals with more servings, you can either enjoy leftovers or reuse parts of the dish for another meal. All of the recipes are designed to be quick and easy, so you can have more leisure time!

Cooking for two might be a bit unfamiliar to you, so I'll share some tips for stocking up on items that you'll use every week and others that you can freeze for future use. To help transition your shopping and planning, you'll want to inventory your pantry first. Having a strategy when you go grocery shopping makes planning healthy meals more effective and reduces food waste.

If you and a loved one have different dietary needs, the good news is that DASH is a healthy plan for just about everyone. The exceptions will be those with celiac disease, gluten intolerance, certain gastrointestinal disorders (including liver disease), or those who require a specific diet for another metabolic disorder. If you are gluten or lactose intolerant, you can still implement most of the DASH principles, making the necessary alterations to the recipes to reflect your specific diet.

### BUILDING YOUR DASH PANTRY

A properly stocked pantry is a secret weapon when it comes to quick and healthy meals. Now is an excellent time to stop procrastinating and reorganize and clean your pantry.

Enlist the assistance of a partner, and you'll be done in no time. Begin by taking everything out, then wiping down the shelves. Toss outdated items in the garbage. If there are items you don't think you'll use up soon, donate them to a local food pantry. You may be surprised to find that many of the things you have on hand fit into DASH recipes.

While you won't be eliminating sodium from your diet, it can be beneficial to reduce it. You probably know that salt is high in sodium, but sodium can lurk in less obvious products in your pantry, as well. Toss or donate the ones high in sodium.

## FOODS TO STOCK

To build your DASH pantry, always have an assortment of shelf-stable staples. Things to keep on hand include rice (arborio, brown, quick-cooking, wild, jasmine, and basmati), whole-wheat and regular pasta (macaroni, linguine, spaghetti, and penne), lentils, beans (black beans, cannelloni beans, and pinto beans), barley, canned goods (tuna, salmon, tomatoes, tomato paste, tomato purée, and fruit), and oats.

Secondly, check your freezer. You'll want to avoid most processed frozen foods, but there are a few items suitable for quick dishes. It's fabulous to have frozen vegetables for times that you don't have fresh. Consider stocking frozen peas, mixed vegetables, butternut squash, bell peppers with onions, shrimp, vacuum-packed fish fillets, and skinless, boneless chicken.

Produce is something that you'll shop for a couple of times a week. I always recommend shopping the sales and specials in the produce section. Generally, the fruits and vegetables on sale are those in season, so they will be budget-friendly and excellent quality. Stores often place items with impending expiration dates on sale. If spinach is buy-one-get-one-free, then today is a good day to buy and cook spinach!

Take a good look at your spice rack, too, because sodium-free spices and herbs add incredible flavor to your recipes. Definitely look for salt-free seasoning blends at the grocery store; this book uses several blends. I like Spice Hunter brand. Many spice blends contain sodium, so scan the ingredient list for salt before popping any in your cart. (You can still use these occasionally in place of salt.) Individual spices such as chili powder, paprika, cumin, coriander, cayenne pepper, black pepper, turmeric, cinnamon, and ground ginger are all great salt-free spices that kick up the flavor of a dish. Fresh herbs and citrus (lemons, limes, oranges) also elevate your meals. For convenience and budget, you'll also want a supply of dried herbs, such as thyme, sage, oregano, parsley, Herbs de Provence, and rosemary.

## WHAT YOU NEED TO KNOW ABOUT VITAMIN K

Vitamin K is needed for the body to produce prothrombin, a protein and clotting factor. Low levels of vitamins K and D have been associated with high blood pressure. The suggested daily intake for vitamin K is 90 micrograms for women and 120 micrograms for men. Leafy green vegetables, such as kale, spinach, Swiss chard, or collards, are not only an excellent addition to your DASH lifestyle but are also great sources of vitamin K. Other sources include soybean and canola oils, Brussels sprouts, broccoli, asparagus, sauerkraut, soybeans, and edamame. Fruits contribute to your daily vitamin K needs as well, with blueberries supplying about 35 percent of daily needs and other fruits providing anywhere from 5 to 25 percent.

It's rare for people to be deficient in vitamin K, and you'll be sure to get an adequate supply following DASH. If you are taking an anticoagulant, you can still consume foods high in vitamin K. You'll want to avoid drastic changes in your diet and check with your doctor regularly.

## Shopping for Two

When you're cooking for two, you'll need a strategy for grocery shopping. Since the recipes that follow are specifically designed for two people, most of the recipes will provide two to three servings.

If you like to shop at the "big box" stores, you need to think about what you'll actually use in a week. Some items (seafood, lean meats, nuts) are often discounted at these stores. You can purchase the larger amount and then break items down into two-serving portions and freeze them in quart-size freezer bags. Big box stores can have a lovely selection of produce and meat, but the quantity can be way too big for a household of two. Plus, there's a lot of temptation there (cue giant boxes of junk food). Save your money, waste less, and buy what you need from a local grocer.

It can be helpful to use a weekly meal plan as the base for your shopping trips. You might consider creating a week's meal plan on Sunday, take an inventory of what you already have in the house, and purchase what you need for the week's recipes. I suggest monthly, weekly, and biweekly shopping runs to stock staple products and ensure high-quality fresh items.

➤ **Monthly**: Check your stock of shelf-stable items such as grains, canned goods, lentils, salt-free spices, nut butters, and frozen foods (fruits, vegetables, veggie burgers, fish, or shrimp).

➤ **Weekly**: Fruits and vegetables (carrots, celery, onions, broccoli, cauliflower, squash, potatoes, apples, melon, grapes, citrus, berries), bread, rolls, low-fat milk, plain Greek yogurt, hummus, light cream cheese, and hard cheeses.

➤ **Biweekly**: More delicate fruits and vegetables (leafy greens, tomatoes, cucumbers, zucchini, pears, bananas), and lean fresh meats.

## REDUCING FOOD WASTE

Americans throw out vast quantities of food every day. According to the Environmental Protection Agency, about 94 percent of that waste ends up in landfills, where it emits methane, a greenhouse gas. Greenhouse gas emission is a growing problem that impacts climate change. You can help reduce your contribution to these landfills by taking a few simple steps. The tips and recipes in this cookbook will help you reduce the food you throw away. By planning shopping trips with food waste in mind, you'll not only be helping improve your health but also the health of the planet.

## DECODING FOOD LABELS

You may already be a label reader, but are you reading labels correctly? Two nutrients you'll want to focus on are sodium and saturated fat. Even though DASH isn't necessarily always a low-salt diet, high-sodium foods should be limited overall. Since your focus is on the whole eating pattern, you'll still be able to choose some higher sodium items once in a while.

Your total sodium intake for the day is going to be around 2300 to 3000 milligrams. This target will help you keep product labels in perspective. While 500 milligrams may seem fairly high for a serving, it is acceptable if your overall sodium intake is low that day. Mostly, you'll want to compare labels. For instance, a surprising source of sodium is bread. Two slices of packaged bread can contain 220 to 300 milligrams of sodium, so compare brands and choose one with less sodium per serving.

Fruits, vegetables, and most fresh meats are low in sodium. When buying frozen vegetables, peruse the label to ensure the product has no added surprises that will increase your daily intake of this mineral. Canned vegetables are higher in sodium, so choose fresh or frozen as often as possible. Since beans are so nutrient-dense, it's okay to choose convenience even though canned beans are higher in sodium than dried. Choose reduced-sodium brands and rinse the beans or vegetables thoroughly. When buying plant-oil spreads, check the saturated fat content and choose brands that have less than two grams per serving. While you don't have to focus on calories, calories still count, and the calories listed are for the serving size specified on the package label.

## Kitchen Equipment

Having the right tools definitely makes cooking more pleasant. There are even a few tools that can help you get more flavor out of ingredients when you're cooking with less salt. Take an inventory of what you already have, then organize a shopping list for some of the items you may want to add so that cooking for two is easier.

### MUST-HAVES

Here are my suggested kitchen equipment must-haves:

2 (1-quart) baking dishes

2 (17-by-11-inch) baking sheets, one rimmed and one flat

2 cutting boards for designated products

2-quart baking dish

4-ounce ramekins

6-cup muffin tin (silicone or nonstick)

Blender

Chef's knife, paring knife, 8-inch utility knife

Colander

Garlic press

High-speed blender

Kitchen shears

Large cast-iron skillet

Large nonstick skillet

Large stockpot

Medium nonstick skillet

Medium saucepan

Parchment paper, aluminum foil,
  wax paper

Pasta pot

Peeler

Pizza pan

Rubber spatulas (3 sizes: large, skinny,
  and mini)

Wooden spoons, metal spatulas, tongs

Zester

### NICE TO HAVE

These tools aren't essential but are nice to have in your kitchen. Several are used in recipes in this book (for example, the slow cooker).

Dutch oven

Glass storage bowls with lids

Immersion blender

Knife sharpener

Manual citrus juicer

Mini 2-cup food processor

Oven–style air fryer

Pizza stone

Salad/herb chopper knife

Silicone baking mats

Silicone lids/splatter guards

Slow cooker

Small broiler pan

Spiralizer

## About the Recipes

The goal of this book is not just to simplify creating DASH meals for two, but also help make healthy cooking less time-consuming and complicated. To that end, most of the recipes use fewer than 10 ingredients. I'll also include tips to modify recipes, swap one ingredient for another, and even to make substitutions when using some packaged products. Nutrition information will be listed under each recipe, too.

Some of the recipes will have an extra serving of some ingredients, which will be incorporated into other recipes. This will introduce you to the "cook once, eat thrice" philosophy that will save you time and reduce food waste.

Recipes are tagged with one or more recipe labels. Since I want eating well to be quick and easy, I included One-Pot (meaning you'll cook the whole dish in just one vessel) and 30 Minutes or Less recipe labels. I also included plant-based recipes (Vegan and Vegetarian), as well as Make-Ahead (to save you time) and Budget-Saver labels to mind your bank account (busting the myth that healthy eating has to cost a fortune).

Whether you enjoy being in the kitchen or not, I know you don't want meal preparation to be complicated. The goal of this book is to help you enjoy life and make adopting a healthy lifestyle easy!

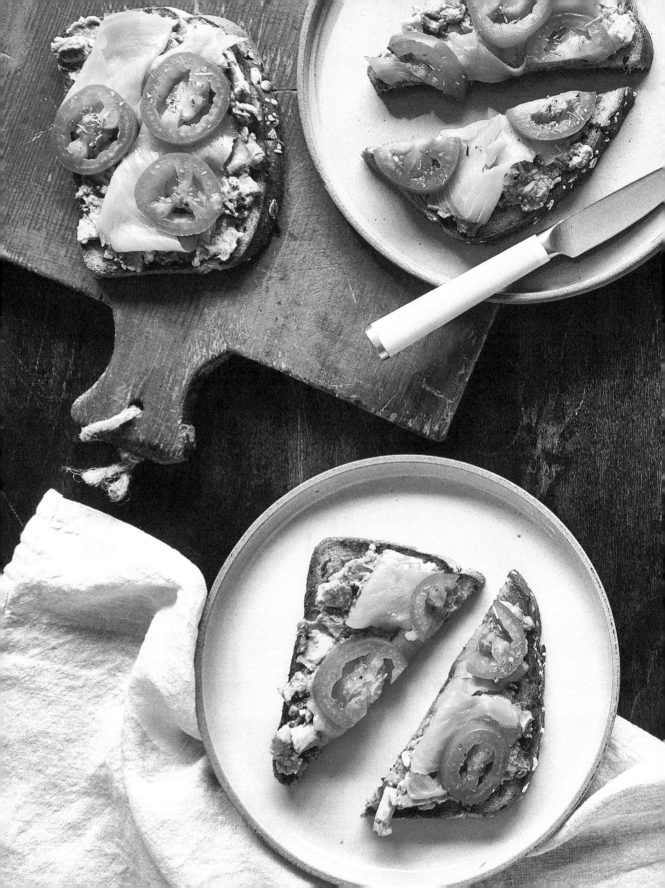

# 2
# BREAKFAST

# Healthy Start Yogurt Bowls

✓ **30 MINUTES OR LESS**
✓ **ONE-POT**
✓ **VEGETARIAN**

**SERVES 2**

**PREP TIME:** 5 MINUTES

2 cups plain low-fat or nonfat Greek yogurt

1 cup fresh or frozen berries

½ cup granola with nuts and seeds

1 teaspoon honey or maple syrup

These simple yogurt bowls are a delicious everyday DASH breakfast. They're wonderful because they include four of the DASH food groups: low-fat dairy, fruit, seeds, and grains. There is a variety of granola on the market. Look for one that has less than 8 grams of sugar per serving and includes both nuts and seeds.

1. Divide the yogurt into two shallow bowls.

2. Arrange half of the berries on the left side of each bowl. Add half of the granola to the right side of each bowl.

3. Drizzle ½ teaspoon of honey or syrup over each bowl and serve.

**SUBSTITUTION TIP:** You can use just about any fruit you like. Pear, banana, and mango are stellar choices. If using dried fruit, use only 2 to 4 tablespoons per bowl to limit sugar.

. . . . . . . . . . . . . . . . . . . . . . . . . . . . . . . . . . . . . . . . . . . . . . . . . .

**Per Serving** Calories: 308; Total fat: 7g; Carbohydrates: 48g; Fiber: 5g; Protein: 16g; Calcium: 484mg; Sodium: 186mg; Potassium: 750mg; Vitamin D: 0mcg; Iron: 1mg; Zinc: 3mg

# On the Run Breakfast Smoothie

**SERVES 2**

**PREP TIME:** 5 MINUTES

1 medium ripe banana

3 tablespoons peanut
  butter powder

1 cup fresh raspberries

1 cup 1 percent milk

1 teaspoon honey

This PB and J smoothie is ideal for days when you're in a rush, or when you just need a light breakfast. The protein-carbohydrate combination is also excellent for exercise recovery after a workout. If you can't find peanut butter powder, add 2 tablespoons of peanut butter instead. Peanut butter has three times the calories of peanut butter powder and provides about the same protein.

1. Put the banana, peanut butter powder, and berries into a blender. Add the milk and honey and blend until smooth, about 1 minute.

2. Pour the smoothie into two glasses and enjoy.

**SUBSTITUTION TIP:** You can substitute strawberries for raspberries if you prefer.

**PREP TIP:** A blender that is at least 500 watts will provide the best results. When making smoothies, put whole ingredients in first, then add the liquid.

. . . . . . . . . . . . . . . . . . . . . . . . . . . . . . . . . . . . . . . . . . . . . . . . .

**Per Serving** Calories: 265; Total fat: 9g; Carbohydrates: 33g; Fiber: 6g; Protein: 9g; Calcium: 164mg; Sodium: 57mg; Potassium: 556mg; Vitamin D: 0mcg; Iron: 1mg; Zinc: 1mg

# Mean Green Morning Juice

**SERVES 2**

**PREP TIME:** 10 MINUTES

2 small Granny Smith
  apples, cored and cut into
  ½-inch pieces or slices

3 cups fresh baby spinach

Juice of 1 lime

2 teaspoons flaxseed

2 ice cubes

This is not a sweet smoothie; the tart apples and lime will wake up your taste buds, and the fresh green color will remind you of spring. It is a breeze getting two to three servings of fruit and veggies into your daily DASH routine when you enjoy this smoothie. Plus, it contains fewer calories per ounce than store-bought juices. This low-calorie, no-sugar-added juice is loaded with vitamins A and C, folic acid, potassium, magnesium, and some iron.

1. Put the apples, spinach, lime juice, and flaxseed into a blender. Add the ice cubes and blend until smooth, about 1 minute. Add water as needed to adjust the texture.

2. Pour the smoothie into two glasses and enjoy!

**VARIATION TIP:** If you enjoy a little spice, add half a teaspoon of turmeric or ground ginger for additional antioxidants.

**STORAGE TIP:** Keep the flaxseed in the refrigerator for up to 6 months or the freezer for a year; this ingredient can go rancid if kept at room temperature.

. . . . . . . . . . . . . . . . . . . . . . . . . . . . . . . . . . . . . . . . . .

**Per Serving** Calories: 118; Total fat: 2g; Carbohydrates: 24g; Fiber: 6g; Protein: 3g; Calcium: 64mg; Sodium: 38mg; Potassium: 477mg; Vitamin D: 0mcg; Iron: 2mg; Zinc: 0mg

# Cottage Cheese Smoothie with Peaches

✓ 30 MINUTES OR LESS
✓ VEGETARIAN

**SERVES 2**

**PREP TIME:** 10 MINUTES

2 peaches, peeled, pitted, and sliced

1 cup low-fat small curd cottage cheese

1 cup 1 percent milk

3 ice cubes

Peach cheesecake in a glass—what is a better way to start your day? Adding low-fat dairy to this luscious smoothie is an effortless way to incorporate food that can lower blood pressure. Cottage cheese is a versatile ingredient that can also be delicious in entrees and even desserts! It adds protein, potassium, and calcium and provides the tart creaminess in this smoothie.

1. Put the peaches, cottage cheese, milk, and ice cubes in a blender and blend until smooth, about 1 minute.

2. Pour into two tall glasses, and garnish with a peach slice, if desired.

**SUBSTITUTION TIP:** You can use drained canned peaches (packed in water or juice) in place of fresh fruit.

**VARIATION TIP:** Try this recipe with mango instead of peaches. They are similar in texture and sweetness, so they provide a nice consistency for the cottage cheese.

. . . . . . . . . . . . . . . . . . . . . . . . . . . . . . . . . . . . . . . . . . . . . . . . .

**Per Serving** Calories: 191; Total fat: 3g; Carbohydrates: 23g; Fiber: 2g; Protein: 19g; Calcium: 230mg; Sodium: 512mg; Potassium: 565mg; Vitamin D: 1mcg; Iron: 1mg; Zinc: 1mg

# Whole-Grain Blueberry Banana Muffins

✔ BUDGET-SAVER
✔ MAKE-AHEAD
✔ VEGETARIAN

**MAKES 6 MUFFINS**

**PREP TIME:** 15 MINUTES
**COOK TIME:** 22 MINUTES

Nonstick cooking spray

2 ripe bananas, mashed

⅓ cup granulated sugar

½ teaspoon pure
  vanilla extract

1 large egg

¼ cup canola oil

1 cup whole-wheat flour

½ cup rolled oats

1 teaspoon baking powder

½ teaspoon
  ground cinnamon

⅛ teaspoon salt

1 cup blueberries

Unlike bakery or coffee shop muffins, homemade muffins are nutritious, low-sugar, high-fiber, and a source of healthy fats. The bananas create a moist sweetness, and the oat and whole-wheat base ensure that one muffin will keep you satiated all morning.

1. Preheat the oven to 350°F. Lightly spray a 6-cup muffin tin with cooking spray.

2. Place the bananas in a medium bowl. Add the sugar and stir well. Add the vanilla extract, egg, and oil and stir well to combine. Set aside.

3. In a separate medium bowl, whisk the flour, oats, baking powder, cinnamon, and salt.

4. Add the dry ingredients to the banana mixture and stir until the flour mixture is just combined. Fold in the blueberries.

5. Spoon the batter evenly into the muffin cups. Bake for 20 to 22 minutes, or until lightly browned.

6. Store in an airtight container in the refrigerator for up to 5 days or freeze for up to 3 months.

**SUBSTITUTION TIP:** You can substitute frozen blueberries for fresh, but they may tint the batter blue.

**VARIATION TIP:** Throw in a half cup of chopped walnuts to add omega-3 fatty acids to the muffins.

. . . . . . . . . . . . . . . . . . . . . . . . . . . . . . . . . . . . . . . . . . . . . . .

**Per Serving (1 muffin)** Calories: 305; Total fat: 11g; Carbohydrates: 47g; Fiber: 5g; Protein: 7g; Calcium: 60mg; Sodium: 66mg; Potassium: 386mg; Vitamin D: 0mcg; Iron: 2mg; Zinc: 1mg

# Maple Quick Oats with Chia & Banana

✔ **30 MINUTES OR LESS**
✔ **ONE-POT**
✔ **VEGETARIAN**

**SERVES 2**

**PREP TIME:** 5 MINUTES
**COOK TIME:** 5 MINUTES

2 cups 1 percent or
  nonfat milk

1 cup quick-cooking oats

1 large banana, sliced

2 teaspoons chia seeds

⅛ teaspoon salt

1 tablespoon pure
  maple syrup

A warm bowl of oatmeal is heart-healthy, comforting, and filling. The fruit is stirred right into the oats, so this dish is like rich banana bread in a bowl. Due to its soluble fiber, oatmeal can also help reduce cholesterol. Making it with milk creates a creamy, rich porridge and also adds protein, which, along with the fiber, will help keep you full until lunch.

1. In a large saucepan, bring the milk to a boil over medium heat.

2. Add the oats and cook for 1 minute, stirring occasionally, until most of the milk is absorbed.

3. Stir the sliced banana, chia seeds, and salt into the oatmeal.

4. Evenly divide the oatmeal into two bowls and drizzle with maple syrup.

**PREP TIP:** You can also make this dish in a microwave, but to avoid spillage, make one portion at a time using a deep bowl. Place 1 cup of oats, 1 teaspoon of chia seeds, and 1 cup of water into a bowl. Microwave for 2 to 2½ minutes, watching it closely. Add the banana to the hot oats and drizzle with maple syrup.

. . . . . . . . . . . . . . . . . . . . . . . . . . . . . . . . . . . . . . . . . . . .

**Per Serving** Calories: 509; Total fat: 9g; Carbohydrates: 87g; Fiber: 11g; Protein: 23g; Calcium: 387mg; Sodium: 286mg; Potassium: 1,008mg; Vitamin D: 2mcg; Iron: 4mg; Zinc: 4mg

# Super Veggie Scramble or Soft Taco

✓ 30 MINUTES OR LESS
✓ ONE-POT
✓ VEGETARIAN

**SERVES 2**

**PREP TIME:** 5 MINUTES
**COOK TIME:** 7 MINUTES

1 tablespoon olive oil

1 medium bell pepper,
  finely chopped

1 small onion,
  finely chopped

2 cups fresh baby spinach,
  finely chopped

3 large eggs

¼ cup 1 percent milk

½ teaspoon paprika

Freshly ground black pepper

1 small avocado, sliced

2 whole-wheat tortillas
  or 2 slices whole-wheat
  toast (optional)

Eggs are high in protein and a good source of vitamin E and choline. Although high in cholesterol, eggs are also a fabulous vehicle for vegetables, like vitamin C–rich peppers, spinach, and avocados. You can use three smaller mixed (yellow, orange, or red) bell peppers instead of one large green pepper for a pop of color. You'll hit three DASH targets with this meal: vegetables, healthy fat, and whole grains (if you include the whole-grain toast or tortilla).

1. Heat the oil in a medium skillet over medium heat.

2. Add the peppers and onion and sauté until the onion is translucent, about 3 minutes. Add the spinach, reduce the heat to low, cover, and cook until the spinach is wilted, about 2 minutes.

3. While the spinach is cooking, in a small bowl, whisk together the eggs, milk, paprika, and a pinch of pepper.

4. Pour the egg mixture over the vegetables in the skillet and stir until the eggs are cooked, about 2 minutes.

5. Divide the eggs between two plates and top with sliced avocado.

6. Serve in a tortilla or with a slice of whole-wheat toast (if using).

**SUBSTITUTION TIP:** Instead of avocado, you can add 2 tablespoons of crumbled feta cheese.

. . . . . . . . . . . . . . . . . . . . . . . . . . . . . . . . . . . . . . . . . .

**Per Serving** Calories: 397; Total fat: 30g; Carbohydrates: 21g; Fiber: 11g; Protein: 16g; Calcium: 140mg; Sodium: 150mg; Potassium: 1019mg; Vitamin D: 2mcg; Iron: 3mg; Zinc: 2mg

# Avocado Toast with Salmon & Tomato

**SERVES 2**

**PREP TIME:** 5 MINUTES
**COOK TIME:** 3 MINUTES

1 large avocado, peeled and pitted

1 teaspoon freshly squeezed lemon juice

4 slices multi-grain bread

3 ounces smoked salmon

2 plum tomatoes, thinly sliced

Salt-free Italian seasoning blend

There is a reason why people are wild about avocado toast. The crunch of the bread and the velvety avocado create an exquisite texture combination in your mouth. Avocado is high in monounsaturated fat, a heart-healthy fat that can help lower your LDL (or "bad" cholesterol). This breakfast also includes salmon, which contains heart-healthy omega-3 fatty acids. A double win! Although delicious, smoked salmon is a higher-sodium item. To reduce sodium, you can use a pouch or can of salmon instead.

1. Put the avocado in a small bowl and mash it lightly with the lemon juice. Set aside.

2. Toast the 4 slices of bread. When toasted, spread each slice with the avocado, dividing it evenly.

3. Top the avocado with smoked salmon, tomato slices, and a sprinkle of seasoning.

4. Cut each slice in half and serve.

**SUBSTITUTION TIP:** Try whole-grain English muffins or bagels instead of bread.

. . . . . . . . . . . . . . . . . . . . . . . . . . . . . . . . . . . . . . . . . . . . . . . .

**Per Serving** Calories: 382; Total fat: 20g; Carbohydrates: 37g; Fiber: 13g; Protein: 19g; Calcium: 80mg; Sodium: 490mg; Potassium: 877mg; Vitamin D: 7mcg; Iron: 2mg; Zinc: 2mg

# Ricotta Toast with Honey & Pistachios

✔ **30 MINUTES OR LESS**
✔ **BUDGET-SAVER**
✔ **ONE-POT**
✔ **VEGETARIAN**

**SERVES 2**

**PREP TIME:** 5 MINUTES
**COOK TIME:** 5 MINUTES

2 slices multi-grain
   seeded bread

¼ cup part-skim
   ricotta cheese

2 tablespoons coarsely
   chopped pistachios

1 teaspoon honey

You may associate ricotta with lasagna and pizza, but this mild, creamy ingredient has many other uses. It's delicious on its own or with fruit, and as you'll see, it makes an unexpectedly delicious topping for toast. Ricotta adds protein, potassium, and calcium to the meal. It's higher in fat than cottage cheese but lower in sodium. When combined with a hint of sweet honey and the buttery crunch of pistachios, ricotta becomes a culinary star.

1. Toast the bread slices until lightly brown and crisp.

2. Spread the toast with ricotta. Evenly divide the chopped nuts between the slices, drizzle them with honey, and serve.

**SUBSTITUTION TIP:** You can use any whole-grain bread for this recipe. Sliced strawberries and chopped walnuts are also an excellent swap for the pistachios and honey.

. . . . . . . . . . . . . . . . . . . . . . . . . . . . . . . . . . . . . . . . . . . . . . .

**Per Serving** Calories: 166; Total fat: 7g; Carbohydrates: 18g; Fiber: 3g; Protein: 9g; Calcium: 119mg; Sodium: 130mg; Potassium: 179mg; Vitamin D: 0mcg; Iron: 1mg; Zinc: 1mg

# Veggie Frittata

✔ **30 MINUTES OR LESS**
✔ **ONE-POT**
✔ **VEGETARIAN**

**SERVES 2**

**PREP TIME:** 10 MINUTES
**COOK TIME:** 10 MINUTES

3 large eggs

½ cup part-skim
  ricotta cheese

Freshly ground
  black pepper

⅛ teaspoon salt

Nonstick cooking spray

1 teaspoon olive oil

1 small zucchini, cut into
  ¼-inch slices

½ cup thinly
  sliced mushrooms

2 tablespoons minced onion

A frittata is a filling breakfast that converts easily into a wonderful lunch or dinner. While it seems fancy, this egg dish is a snap to make and a joy to eat. Add a slice of toast and some fruit, and you've got a full DASH meal in minutes.

1. In a medium bowl, beat the eggs. Fold in the ricotta and whisk until the eggs are foamy. Add a pinch of pepper and the salt.

2. Spray an 8-to-10-inch oven-safe (e.g., cast-iron) skillet with cooking spray. Add the oil and heat it over medium heat for 1 to 2 minutes.

3. Add the zucchini, mushrooms, and onion and cook for 3 to 4 minutes, until tender. While the vegetables are cooking, turn on the broiler and set it to 450°F.

4. Pour the egg mixture over the vegetables, shaking the skillet until the eggs are evenly dispersed. Turn the heat to low, and allow the eggs to cook, untouched, for 2 minutes.

5. Transfer the skillet to the oven and broil on high for 1 to 2 minutes, until lightly browned.

6. Remove the skillet from the oven. Use a metal spatula to loosen the frittata from the skillet, place a large plate over the skillet, then carefully invert the frittata onto the plate, and serve.

**STORAGE TIP:** You can store leftovers in the refrigerator for two days and reheat in the microwave for 30 to 60 seconds, or on the stove in a pan over low heat for 4 to 5 minutes.

. . . . . . . . . . . . . . . . . . . . . . . . . . . . . . . . . . . . . . . . . . . . .

**Per Serving** Calories: 232; Total fat: 15g; Carbohydrates: 7g; Fiber: 1g; Protein: 18g; Calcium: 223mg; Sodium: 329mg; Potassium: 405mg; Vitamin D: 2mcg; Iron: 2mg; Zinc: 2mg

# Superfood Egg Cups

✔ **30 MINUTES OR LESS**
✔ **MAKE-AHEAD**
✔ **ONE-POT**
✔ **VEGETARIAN**

**SERVES 3**

**PREP TIME:** 10 MINUTES
**COOK TIME:** 14 MINUTES

Nonstick cooking spray

6 large eggs

3 tablespoons
 1 percent milk

Freshly ground
 black pepper

⅓ cup fresh baby
 spinach, chopped

¼ cup bell pepper, minced

¼ cup shredded
 Swiss cheese

These colorful, versatile egg cups are quick, easy, and can be made ahead for a perfect grab-and-go meal. These muffin-size frittatas can be eaten plain or sandwiched between the halves of a whole-grain English muffin for a more substantial meal. Cheese is high in saturated fat and sodium but so flavorful that a little goes a long way. You will not need to add salt with a sprinkle of rich cheese, which makes the meal healthier, as well.

1.  Preheat the oven to 350°F. Spray a 6-cup muffin tin (metal or silicone) with nonstick cooking spray.

2.  In a medium bowl, whisk the eggs with the milk. Season with pepper and set aside.

3.  Divide the vegetables and cheese evenly between the muffin cups. Pour the egg mixture into the muffin cups, filling them about two-thirds full.

4.  Bake the egg cups for 10 to 14 minutes, until firm but not overly browned.

5.  Let them cool for 5 minutes, then remove them from the muffin tin and serve.

**VARIATION TIP:** Other great combinations include goat cheese with asparagus, spinach and feta, peppers with a sharp cheddar or pepper jack cheese, and onions and chopped tomatoes with fontina. You can also make each cup different!

**STORAGE TIP:** Store in an airtight freezer bag in the freezer for up to a month.

. . . . . . . . . . . . . . . . . . . . . . . . . . . . . . . . . . . . . . . . . . . . .

**Per Serving** Calories: 188; Total fat: 12g; Carbohydrates: 3g; Fiber: 0g; Protein: 16g; Calcium: 150mg; Sodium: 158mg; Potassium: 202mg; Vitamin D: 2mcg; Iron: 2mg; Zinc: 2mg

# Sweet Potato Hash

✔ ONE-POT
✔ VEGAN

**SERVES 2**

**PREP TIME:** 15 MINUTES
**COOK TIME:** 20 MINUTES

1 tablespoon olive oil

1 small green bell pepper, diced

3 tablespoons diced sweet onion

2 medium sweet potatoes, peeled and diced

1 teaspoon smoked paprika

1 garlic clove, pressed or minced

Freshly ground black pepper

This hearty dish is ideal for making on a weekend when you have a little more time to relax. Sweet potatoes take the place of the more common white potato in this onion and pepper–studded hash. Sweet potatoes are a good source of fiber, vitamins C and A, and potassium. They're flavorful enough to provide an excellent base for this savory, filling, and low-calorie breakfast treat.

1. Heat the oil in a large skillet over medium heat. Add the peppers and onion and cook until the onion is translucent, about 3 minutes.

2. Add the diced sweet potatoes and stir until the vegetables are evenly mixed. Add the paprika and garlic. Cover and cook over low to medium heat with minimal stirring, allowing the onions to caramelize and the potatoes to brown, for about 10 minutes.

3. Continue cooking an additional 4 to 7 minutes, or until the potatoes are tender.

4. Season with freshly ground black pepper and serve.

**VARIATION TIP:** For extra protein and fiber, add ½ cup canned black beans, drained and rinsed, in step 3. You can also add an egg or two to this and treat the hash as a side dish.

**STORAGE TIP:** Store leftovers in the refrigerator for up to 4 days.

· · · · · · · · · · · · · · · · · · · · · · · · · · · · · · · · · · · · · · · · · · · · · ·

**Per Serving** Calories: 190; Total fat: 7g; Carbohydrates: 30g; Fiber: 5g; Protein: 3g; Calcium: 52mg; Sodium: 74mg; Potassium: 557mg; Vitamin D: 0mcg; Iron: 1mg; Zinc: 1mg

# Ricotta French Toast with Sliced Pears

✓ **30 MINUTES OR LESS**
✓ **ONE-POT**
✓ **VEGETARIAN**

**SERVES 2**

**PREP TIME:** 10 MINUTES
**COOK TIME:** 12 MINUTES

1 large Anjou pear, peeled, cored, and thinly sliced

Juice of ½ lemon

2 large eggs

½ cup 1 percent milk

¼ cup part-skim ricotta

¼ teaspoon nutmeg

Nonstick cooking spray

4 slices crusty whole-grain bread, 1 inch thick

1 tablespoon honey

This makes a lovely special occasion breakfast or brunch for two, or you can double or triple the recipe for company. The ricotta adds body and flavor to the French toast mixture, as well as extra protein. The pears offer a distinctive sweetness and go beautifully with the ricotta, but you can also substitute fresh strawberries, raspberries, or blueberries.

1. Put the pear slices and the lemon juice into a small bowl, toss lightly, and set aside.

2. In a medium bowl, whisk the eggs. Add the milk and ricotta and whisk well. Then add the nutmeg and stir to combine.

3. Heat a large nonstick skillet coated with cooking spray over medium heat. Dip 2 slices of bread into the egg mixture, turning to coat thoroughly. Transfer the bread to the skillet and cook until each side is lightly browned, 2 to 3 minutes per side. Transfer the bread to a plate and set aside. Repeat with the remaining 2 slices of bread.

4. Serve the French toast topped with sliced pears and a drizzle of honey.

**VARIATION TIP:** For French toast, firm, crusty bread works best. Try French, Italian, or whole-grain ciabatta. If you don't have fresh pears, you can also use drained canned pears packed in their own juice.

. . . . . . . . . . . . . . . . . . . . . . . . . . . . . . . . . . . . . . . . . . . . . . . . . . . . . . . . . . .

**Per Serving** Calories: 384; Total fat: 10g; Carbohydrates: 54g; Fiber: 7g; Protein: 19g; Calcium: 256mg; Sodium: 328mg; Potassium: 475mg; Vitamin D: 2mcg; Iron: 3mg; Zinc: 2mg

# Sleeping-In Overnight Oats

✔ ONE-POT

✔ VEGETARIAN

**SERVES 2**

**PREP TIME:** 10 MINUTES,
PLUS OVERNIGHT

⅔ cup rolled oats

1 tablespoon chia seeds

2 tablespoons
 peanut butter

1 cup 1 percent milk

1 cup whole blueberries

2 teaspoons
 honey (optional)

This recipe is perfect for hectic mornings or days when you want to hit the snooze button and still have a nutritious breakfast ready to eat. The best container to use is a small (pint-size) mason jar, but a covered bowl works, too. Overnight oats are similar to muesli and are served chilled so they can be made days ahead, and they cover a lot of DASH nutrition bases. Blueberries are my favorite fruit for oats, but you can also use sliced strawberries or mango.

1. Evenly divide the oats, seeds, and peanut butter between two small mason jars. Pour a ¼ cup of milk into each jar and stir until combined. Evenly divide the remaining milk between the jars and stir until thoroughly mixed.

2. Divide the berries evenly between both jars, put the lids on tightly, and refrigerate overnight.

3. Enjoy the oats the next morning with a drizzle of honey on top (if using).

**VARIATION TIP:** You can omit the chia seeds, but they give the oats a nice pudding-like texture. If you do not use the chia seeds, reduce the milk to ¾ cup.

. . . . . . . . . . . . . . . . . . . . . . . . . . . . . . . . . . . . . . . . . . . . . . . . . . . . . . .

**Per Serving** Calories: 427; Total fat: 15g; Carbohydrates: 58g; Fiber: 11g; Protein: 18g; Calcium: 238mg; Sodium: 59mg; Potassium: 582mg; Vitamin D: 1mcg; Iron: 3mg; Zinc: 3mg

# Cinnamon Stuffed Sweet Potatoes

✔ ONE-POT

✔ VEGAN

**SERVES 2**

**PREP TIME:** 5 MINUTES
**COOK TIME:** 45 MINUTES

2 large sweet potatoes

4 tablespoons
 peanut butter

½ teaspoon
 ground cinnamon

¼ cup pecans, chopped

You may have never thought about eating a sweet potato for breakfast, but you should! They are fiber-rich and full of beta carotene and other antioxidants. Topped with nut butter, chopped nuts for texture, and cinnamon, these sweet potatoes are almost as indulgent as a sweet roll.

1. Preheat the oven to 400°F.

2. Wash and scrub the potatoes, then cut a 3-inch slit lengthwise into the top of each potato.

3. Place the potatoes directly on the top oven rack and bake for 45 minutes or until soft.

4. Once baked, open each potato and top each with half of the peanut butter, cinnamon, and pecans. Serve warm.

**VARIATION TIP:** Instead of cinnamon and nuts, try nutmeg and raisins or ground cloves with dried cranberries.

**PREP TIP:** To cut down on prep time, you can bake the potatoes ahead of time, store them in the refrigerator, and then reheat them for 2 minutes in the microwave or 10 to 15 minutes in a conventional oven.

. . . . . . . . . . . . . . . . . . . . . . . . . . . . . . . . . . . . . . . . . . . . . . .

**Per Serving** Calories: 399; Total fat: 26g; Carbohydrates: 36g; Fiber: 7g; Protein: 10g; Calcium: 71mg; Sodium: 77mg; Potassium: 675mg; Vitamin D: 0mcg; Iron: 2mg; Zinc: 2mg

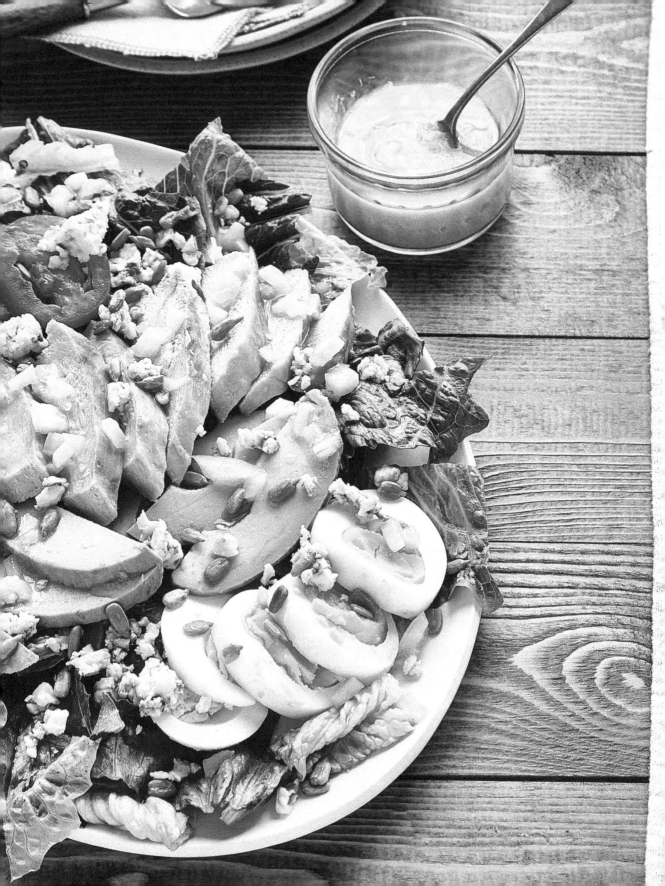

# 3
# SOUPS AND SALADS

# Bibb Lettuce with Beets, Pears & Goat Cheese

✓ **30 MINUTES OR LESS**
✓ **ONE-POT**
✓ **VEGETARIAN**

**SERVES 2**

**PREP TIME:** 10 MINUTES

### For the Salad

1 small head Bibb lettuce, torn into bite-size pieces

2 ripe pears, cored and thinly sliced

3 ounces canned beets, sliced or diced

2 ounces crumbled goat cheese

### For the Dressing

2 tablespoons olive oil

2 teaspoons white wine vinegar

¼ teaspoon honey

2 tablespoons freshly squeezed orange juice

Freshly ground black pepper

Bibb lettuce, also called butter lettuce, is tender, slightly sweet, and delicious. It's a perfect choice when cooking for two because you can usually find a smaller head of Bibb lettuce, and it stays fresh longer than other types. Goat cheese adds a unique tart flavor and oomph to this salad. Serve the salad as a side dish for beef or chicken, such as the 50-50 Burgers with Caramelized Onions (page 151), or pair it with a serving of fruit.

## To Make the Salad

1. Divide the lettuce between two salad plates (about 1½ cups each).

2. Top with the pear slices, beets, and goat cheese.

## To Make the Dressing

3. In a small bowl, whisk together the olive oil, vinegar, honey, and orange juice until blended. Season to taste with the pepper.

4. Drizzle the dressing over the salads and serve immediately.

**SUBSTITUTION TIP:** Apples also work in place of the pears. If you don't have white wine vinegar, you can use balsamic vinegar or 1 teaspoon of Dijon mustard.

**STORAGE TIP:** Leftover beets can be stored in the refrigerator for a week.

. . . . . . . . . . . . . . . . . . . . . . . . . . . . . . . . . . . . . . . . . . . . . . . . .

**Per Serving** Calories: 331; Total fat: 20g; Carbohydrates: 34g; Fiber: 7g; Protein: 7g; Calcium: 93mg; Sodium: 220mg; Potassium: 501mg; Vitamin D: 0mcg; Iron: 3mg; Zinc: 1mg

# Fruit Salad with Honey-Drizzled Ricotta

**SERVES 2**

**PREP TIME:** 15 MINUTES

2 medium crisp apples
(Gala, Fuji, or Honeycrisp),
cored and cut
into ½-inch dice

1 small mango, cut into
½-inch pieces

1 cup blueberries

1 large banana, sliced

1 lime, quartered

1 cup part-skim
ricotta cheese

2 teaspoons honey

2 fresh mint sprigs, for
garnish (optional)

This fruit salad is a good source of potassium and vitamin C and becomes a light meal when paired with ricotta. It's lovely to serve for brunch, as a light breakfast, as a side dish with lunch, or as a dessert. You can use strawberries or melon instead of the blueberries or mango. This salad is best served fresh but can be stored in the refrigerator for up to two days.

1. Put the apples, mango, blueberries, and banana in a small bowl.

2. Squeeze the juice of two lime wedges over the fruit and gently toss with a large spoon.

3. Evenly divide the ricotta between two small bowls and drizzle honey over the ricotta. Spoon the fruit over the ricotta and garnish each bowl with a lime wedge and a fresh mint sprig (if using).

**SUBSTITUTION TIP:** Low-fat cottage cheese can be substituted for the ricotta cheese.

**PREP TIP:** Slice the banana last, so it doesn't brown, or leave it out if storing the salad.

. . . . . . . . . . . . . . . . . . . . . . . . . . . . . . . . . . . . . . . . . . . . . . . . . . .

**Per Serving** Calories: 500; Total fat: 11g; Carbohydrates: 89g; Fiber: 10g; Protein: 17g; Calcium: 379mg; Sodium: 128mg; Potassium: 953mg; Vitamin D: 0mcg; Iron: 1mg; Zinc: 2mg

# Caprese Tomato Salad

✔ **30 MINUTES OR LESS**
✔ **ONE-POT**
✔ **VEGETARIAN**

**SERVES 2**

**PREP TIME:** 15 MINUTES

### For the Salad

6 plum tomatoes, cut into ¼-inch slices

Pinch salt

Fresh basil, about 15 large leaves, thinly sliced

2 ounces fresh mozzarella balls, sliced

### For the Dressing

3 tablespoons extra-virgin olive oil

1 tablespoon balsamic vinegar

Freshly ground black pepper

This classic salad will brighten your day with its fresh and bold flavor. It pairs well with a baked fish dinner like the Baked Haddock with Peppers & Eggplant (page 99) or a half sandwich at lunchtime. Any kind of tomato will do here, but the secret to this salad is using ripe, juicy, sweet ones, preferably warm from the sun in your own garden. You can prep the tomatoes and basil ahead and wait to add the dressing until just before you serve it.

### To Make the Salad

1. Arrange the tomato slices on a small platter. Sprinkle with a pinch of salt.

2. Top with the basil leaves and the mozzarella.

### To Make the Dressing

3. In a small bowl, whisk the olive oil and vinegar. Pour the dressing over the tomatoes and cheese.

4. Season the salad with pepper and serve.

**VARIATION TIP:** If you want to make this into a snack or appetizer, you can substitute cherry tomatoes and skewer two tomatoes on a toothpick with a basil leaf and half of a mozzarella ball. Drizzle with dressing.

. . . . . . . . . . . . . . . . . . . . . . . . . . . . . . . . . . . . . . . . . . . . . . . . .

**Per Serving** Calories: 305; Total fat: 27g; Carbohydrates: 9g; Fiber: 2g; Protein: 8g; Calcium: 171mg; Sodium: 267mg; Potassium: 483mg; Vitamin D: 0mcg; Iron: 1mg; Zinc: 1mg

# Greek Orzo Salad with Cucumbers, Tomato & Feta

✔ ONE-POT
✔ VEGETARIAN

**SERVES 3**

**PREP TIME:** 15 MINUTES, PLUS 20 MINUTES TO COOL
**COOK TIME:** 9 MINUTES

⅓ cup orzo, uncooked

2 tablespoons extra-virgin olive oil

1 tablespoon freshly squeezed lemon juice

1 garlic clove, pressed or minced

Pinch freshly ground black pepper

1 small English cucumber, peeled, sliced, and quartered

½ pint grape tomatoes, halved

¼ cup chopped pitted kalamata olives

3 tablespoons chopped parsley

2 ounces reduced-fat feta cheese, crumbled

This traditional Greek combination provides a refreshing, light lunch or side dish any time of the year. It's a great salad to take to picnics or potlucks and can easily be doubled. Make the orzo ahead, since this salad tastes best after it is refrigerated for at least 3 hours, or overnight. The feta and olives add sodium to the dish, so you don't need added salt. The olives offer healthy fat, too. If you want to lower the sodium even further, you can use less feta.

1. Fill a medium saucepan three-quarters full of water and bring it to a boil over high heat. Cook the orzo al dente (for about 9 minutes or according to package instructions), drain it, and allow it to cool for about 20 minutes.

2. While the orzo cooks, mix the oil, lemon juice, garlic, and pepper in a small bowl and set aside.

3. Put the cooled orzo in a medium bowl. Add the cucumbers, tomatoes, olives, and parsley.

4. Drizzle the dressing over the salad and toss gently until combined. Top with the crumbled feta.

5. Season with additional pepper, if desired, and serve.

**INGREDIENT TIP:** You can use both red and yellow tomatoes to brighten the color of the salad and add flavor.

**STORAGE TIP:** This salad can be stored in the refrigerator for up to four days.

. . . . . . . . . . . . . . . . . . . . . . . . . . . . . . . . . . . . . . . . . . . . .

**Per Serving** Calories: 232; Total fat: 14g; Carbohydrates: 21g; Fiber: 2g; Protein: 5g; Calcium: 123mg; Sodium: 262mg; Potassium: 189mg; Vitamin D: 0mcg; Iron: 1mg; Zinc: 1mg

# Field Greens with Artichoke Hearts & Roasted Peppers

✓ **VEGAN**

**SERVES 2 TO 3**

**PREP TIME:** 15 MINUTES
**COOK TIME:** 20 MINUTES

### For the Salad

5 mini mixed bell
  peppers, halved

¼ cup olive oil, divided

3 cups mixed field greens or
  spring mix salad

1 (8-ounce) jar of artichoke
  hearts (about 6), drained
  and quartered

½ cup chopped walnuts

### For the Dressing

5 teaspoons avocado oil

2 teaspoons white
  wine vinegar

¼ teaspoon sugar

Salads are an ideal way to bump up your DASH vegetable intake. They are quick to prep, and you can layer a variety of veggies into them. This salad has a Mediterranean flair with roasted peppers, artichokes, and healthy fats. Make sure to choose a low-sodium jar of artichoke hearts, as brands vary.

## To Make the Salad

1. Preheat the oven to 450°F. Line a baking sheet with parchment paper.

2. Place the peppers on the baking sheet, brush them with olive oil, and roast for 20 minutes, or until slightly charred.

3. Once the peppers have cooled slightly, chop them coarsely.

4. Arrange the greens onto a plate. Add the artichoke hearts on one-third of the plate, then the peppers on another third, and finally the walnuts on the last third.

## To Make the Dressing

5. In a small bowl, stir together the oil, vinegar, and sugar, blending well. Pour the dressing over the salad and serve.

**VARIATION TIP:** Add a ½ cup of chopped cooked chicken, cooked shrimp, or lentils to add protein.

. . . . . . . . . . . . . . . . . . . . . . . . . . . . . . . . . . . . . . . . . . . . .

**Per Serving** Calories: 645; Total fat: 58g; Carbohydrates: 29g; Fiber: 10g; Protein: 11g; Calcium: 114mg; Sodium: 89mg; Potassium: 1082mg; Vitamin D: 0mcg; Iron: 3mg; Zinc: 2mg

# DASH-Style Cobb Salad

✔ ONE-POT

**SERVES 2**

**PREP TIME:** 20 MINUTES
**COOK TIME:** 15 MINUTES

1 (6-ounce) skinless, boneless chicken breast

Zest and juice of 1 lemon

2 tablespoons white wine vinegar

1 tablespoon extra-virgin olive oil

1 tablespoon sweet onion, minced

½ teaspoon Dijon mustard

1 head romaine lettuce, roughly chopped

1 large hardboiled egg, sliced

4 plum tomatoes, sliced

1 avocado, thinly sliced

1 ounce blue cheese crumbles

1 tablespoon roasted sunflower seeds

A traditional Cobb salad includes bacon and blue cheese, both high in fat and sodium. To make this recipe DASH-friendly, I've replaced the bacon with sunflower seeds and halved the blue cheese, which still adds a wonderful flavor to the salad. This is also an excellent main-dish salad to make when you have leftover cooked chicken.

1. To poach the chicken, fill a large saucepan three-quarters full of water and bring it to a boil over high heat. Add the zest or rind from half of the lemon to the water. Add the chicken, reduce the heat to low, cover, and simmer for about 10 minutes. The chicken should be opaque and white in the center. If it's showing any pink, continue simmering for another 5 minutes. Remove the saucepan from the heat and take the chicken out to cool.

2. While the chicken is cooking, mix the dressing. Combine the vinegar, lemon juice, oil, onion, and mustard in a small bowl or jar and mix thoroughly.

3. Divide the lettuce between two plates and top it with the egg, tomato, and avocado slices.

4. Cut the chicken into ⅛-inch thick slices and add it to the salads. Drizzle the salads with the dressing, top them with blue cheese crumbles and sunflower seeds, and serve.

**INGREDIENT TIP:** You can find cubed frozen avocado at some grocery stores. Defrost and use a few pieces to save a little prep time.

. . . . . . . . . . . . . . . . . . . . . . . . . . . . . . . . . . . . . . . .

**Per Serving** Calories: 542; Total fat: 34g; Carbohydrates: 31g; Fiber: 17g; Protein: 35g; Calcium: 232mg; Sodium: 287mg; Potassium: 1924mg; Vitamin D: 1mcg; Iron: 5mg; Zinc: 3mg

# High Protein Spring Mix with Tuna & Egg

✔ **30 MINUTES OR LESS**

✔ **ONE-POT**

**SERVES 2**

**PREP TIME:** 15 MINUTES

2 (2.6-ounce) pouches of albacore tuna

2 large hardboiled eggs, chopped

¼ cup chopped celery

2 tablespoons minced onion

2 tablespoons plain Greek yogurt

1 tablespoon mayonnaise

¼ teaspoon dried dill

4 cups spring mix or other salad greens

1 cup grape tomatoes, halved

½ cup finely chopped yellow bell peppers

1 tablespoon extra-virgin olive oil

1 tablespoon apple cider vinegar

This salad is a protein powerhouse, boasting more than 20 grams per serving. It also helps you meet your twice-a-week seafood goal. Tuna provides heart-healthy omega-3 fatty acids and is conveniently available in pouches and cans. Check the sodium content on the tuna because it varies between brands. If you're short on time, you can skip mixing the tuna with the eggs and yogurt dressing. Feel free to substitute romaine or Bibb lettuce for the spring mix.

1. In a medium bowl, mix the tuna, eggs, celery, onion, yogurt, mayonnaise, and dill until well combined.

2. Divide the spring mix between two plates. Add half of the tomatoes and peppers to each plate and dress the salads with oil and vinegar.

3. Top each of the salads with a large scoop of the tuna mixture and serve.

**INGREDIENT TIP:** You can add a pinch of sugar to tame the acidity of the vinegar.

. . . . . . . . . . . . . . . . . . . . . . . . . . . . . . . . . . . . . . . . . . . . . . . . . . . .

**Per Serving** Calories: 370; Total fat: 20g; Carbohydrates: 23g; Fiber: 4g; Protein: 27g; Calcium: 134mg; Sodium: 432mg; Potassium: 881mg; Vitamin D: 2mcg; Iron: 3mg; Zinc: 2mg

# Arugula Salad with Tuna & Roasted Peppers

✔ ONE-POT

**SERVES 2**

**PREP TIME:** 15 MINUTES
**COOK TIME:** 21 MINUTES

2 tablespoons plus
 1 teaspoon olive
 oil, divided

2 tablespoons
 balsamic vinegar

Juice of 1½ lemons, divided

2 tuna steaks
 (4 to 6 ounces each)

4 to 6 mini bell
 peppers, seeded and
 halved lengthwise

4 cups arugula

¼ cup fresh basil, chopped

Freshly ground
 black pepper

1 mango, diced

Lemon quarters, for garnish

Arugula is a peppery, tender salad green. It works well as a bed for beef or a tuna-steak salad. The sweet, juicy mango balances the slight bitterness of the greens and, combined with the roasted peppers, offers flavor and substance to the salad, allowing you to use less dressing.

1. Preheat the grill to 450°F.

2. Mix 1 tablespoon of the olive oil, the balsamic vinegar, and the juice of half a lemon in a shallow bowl. Add the tuna to the bowl and marinate it while the peppers cook.

3. Place the peppers on a small grill pan, then put it on the hot grill. Grill for 10 to 15 minutes, or until the peppers are slightly charred, turning occasionally. Transfer them to a small bowl. Using kitchen shears, chop the peppers into large pieces. Add 1 teaspoon of olive oil and set aside to cool.

4. Place the tuna steaks on the hot grill and grill for 3 minutes per side for medium doneness (discard the marinade). Remove the fish from the grill and cut each steak into ¼-inch slices. Cover the tuna with foil to keep it warm.

5. If you do not have a grill, roast the peppers on a baking sheet in a 450°F oven for 25 to 40 minutes, turning them halfway through the cooking time. Cook the tuna in a large nonstick skillet over medium-high heat, 2 to 3 minutes per side.

**CONTINUED** ▶

6. In a medium bowl, toss together the arugula and basil. In a small bowl, mix together the remaining olive oil with the remaining lemon juice. Pour the mixture over the salad and toss to coat.

7. Divide the arugula mixture between two plates. Season to taste with pepper. Top with the roasted peppers, mango and tuna slices. Garnish with a lemon quarter, if desired.

**VARIATION TIP:** For a savory salad, add 1 ounce of crumbled feta cheese and sliced olives instead of the mango.

**INGREDIENT TIP:** You can use frozen mango cubes if you don't have fresh. Be sure to defrost them first.

. . . . . . . . . . . . . . . . . . . . . . . . . . . . . . . . . . . . . . . . . . . . . . .

**Per Serving** Calories: 511; Total fat: 23g; Carbohydrates: 50g; Fiber: 6g; Protein: 32g; Calcium: 134mg; Sodium: 67mg; Potassium: 1271mg; Vitamin D: 6mcg; Iron: 4mg; Zinc: 2mg

# Bold Bean Shrimp Fiesta Salad

✔ **30 MINUTES OR LESS**
✔ **MAKE-AHEAD**
✔ **ONE-POT**

**SERVES 2**

**PREP TIME:** 20 MINUTES

2 cups frozen corn, thawed

1 cup canned black beans, drained and rinsed

1 cup chopped cooked shrimp

1 cup halved grape tomatoes

1 jalapeño pepper, seeded and diced

2 tablespoons diced red onion

Juice of 2 limes

¼ cup chopped fresh cilantro

1½ tablespoons olive oil

⅛ teaspoon salt

Pinch freshly ground black pepper

Canned beans are so convenient and healthy, they should always be on your pantry shelf. Loaded with fiber and B vitamins, these nutrition powerhouses are also filling and a good source of protein. Make sure to rinse the beans, as it removes up to 40 percent of the sodium. If you don't have frozen corn, you can also use drained, low-sodium canned corn. This one-bowl salad can be eaten as-is or used as a topping on a green salad mix.

1. In a medium bowl, combine the corn, beans, shrimp, tomatoes, jalapeño, and onion.

2. In a small bowl or jar, mix the lime juice, cilantro, olive oil, salt, and pepper.

3. Add the dressing to the corn and bean mixture, toss until combined, and serve.

**SUBSTITUTION TIP:** If you're not into spicy food, you can substitute 3 tablespoons of diced bell pepper for the jalapeño. You can also use bottled lime juice instead of fresh limes and chopped chicken instead of shrimp. To make this extra-festive, serve it in half of a pitted avocado.

**PREP TIP:** Roll the lime on the counter before cutting it in half to juice it easier.

. . . . . . . . . . . . . . . . . . . . . . . . . . . . . . . . . . . . . . . . . . . . . . . . . . . .

**Per Serving** Calories: 422; Total fat: 13g; Carbohydrates: 68g; Fiber: 14g; Protein: 19g; Calcium: 68mg; Sodium: 379mg; Potassium: 998mg; Vitamin D: 0mcg; Iron: 3mg; Zinc: 3mg

# Salmon-Topped Spinach Salad with Avocado

✔ 30 MINUTES OR LESS

**SERVES 2**

**PREP TIME:** 20 MINUTES
**COOK TIME:** 10 MINUTES

2 tablespoons avocado oil

Juice of 1 lime

1 tablespoon plus ½ teaspoon mesquite salt-free seasoning blend (or any salt-free seasoning), divided

2 salmon fillets (4 ounces each)

3 cups fresh baby spinach, washed and stemmed

¼ cup dried cranberries

1½ tablespoons sunflower seeds

1 avocado, sliced

Salmon is a heart-healthy fatty fish that is superb grilled or baked. It cooks quickly, so it makes for a simple, quick lunch or dinner. Avocados and sunflower seeds are also sources of healthy monounsaturated fats, which keeps this main-dish salad satisfying. I like to make this recipe in an air fryer, but you can also easily bake it in the oven (see tip).

1. Preheat an oven-style air fryer to 350°F, on the air-fry setting.

2. In a small jar or bowl, mix the avocado oil, lime juice, and ½ teaspoon of the mesquite seasoning. Set aside.

3. Rub both sides of each salmon fillet with the remaining mesquite seasoning and air-fry for 10 minutes.

4. While the salmon is air-frying, in a medium bowl, toss the spinach with the cranberries and sunflower seeds. Drizzle the salad with the dressing and toss to combine.

5. Divide the spinach mixture between two plates. Top each salad with the avocado and the salmon and serve.

**COOKING TIP:** If you don't have an air fryer, you can bake the salmon for 20 minutes in a conventional oven pre-heated to 400°F.

. . . . . . . . . . . . . . . . . . . . . . . . . . . . . . . . . . . . . . . . . . . . . .

**Per Serving** Calories: 568; Total fat: 40g; Carbohydrates: 29g; Fiber: 11g; Protein: 28g; Calcium: 84mg; Sodium: 90mg; Potassium: 1415mg; Vitamin D: 7mcg; Iron: 3mg; Zinc: 2mg

# Moroccan-Inspired Lentil Soup

✔ ONE-POT
✔ VEGETARIAN

**SERVES 4**

**PREP TIME:** 10 MINUTES
**COOK TIME:** 31 MINUTES

1 cup dried green lentils

1 tablespoon olive oil

1 garlic clove, pressed or minced

½ large sweet onion, finely chopped

¾ cup finely chopped carrots

1 red or yellow pepper, finely chopped

4 cups low-sodium vegetable broth

2 tablespoons Moroccan salt-free seasoning blend

¼ cup plain Greek nonfat yogurt, for garnish

If you are unfamiliar with Moroccan cuisine, this unassuming soup will be a taste revelation. Spices from this region of the world usually include chili powder, coriander, garlic, paprika, cinnamon, cumin, and ginger. This spice blend gives food a sweet but earthy flavor, especially legumes, which seem to pick up all the glorious nuances of the spices. Lentils are high in protein (about 18 grams per cup) and fiber and are the ideal base for this comforting, meatless meal.

1. Thoroughly rinse the lentils using a colander or a strainer. Set aside.

2. Heat the olive oil in a Dutch oven over medium-low heat until hot. Add the garlic, onions, carrots, and pepper and sauté until the onion is translucent, 5 to 6 minutes.

3. Add the broth, lentils, and seasoning, then stir and bring to a boil. Once boiling, reduce the heat to low, cover, and simmer for 25 minutes.

4. Serve this soup garnished with yogurt.

**SUBSTITUTION TIP:** Any type of lentils can be used in this recipe: Red, brown, or French lentils are all great options.

**STORAGE TIP:** Store in the refrigerator in an airtight container for up to 3 days or freeze for up to a month.

. . . . . . . . . . . . . . . . . . . . . . . . . . . . . . . . . . . . . . . . . . . . .

**Per Serving** Calories: 230; Total fat: 4g; Carbohydrates: 38g; Fiber: 7g; Protein: 13g; Calcium: 36mg; Sodium: 21mg; Potassium: 531mg; Vitamin D: 0mcg; Iron: 3mg; Zinc: 2mg

# White Bean Soup with Chicken & Spinach

✔ **ONE-POT**

**SERVES 3**

**PREP TIME:** 15 MINUTES
**COOK TIME:** 37 MINUTES

2 teaspoons olive oil

½ cup diced sweet onion

½ cup diced carrots

1½ teaspoons salt-free Italian spice blend

1 tablespoon tomato paste

1 (15-ounce) can cannellini beans, drained and rinsed

1 cup diced cooked chicken breast

4 cups low-sodium chicken broth

1 (6-ounce) bag fresh baby spinach, chopped

1 teaspoon grated Parmesan cheese, for garnish

Freshly ground black pepper

If you have leftover meat or veggies in your refrigerator, soup is a great recipe choice. This hearty creation might remind you of Minestrone, a classic Italian dish. It uses buttery cannellini beans, which are large, white kidney beans high in fiber and B vitamins. This bean is incredibly versatile and is often used in pasta dishes, dips, or mixed with vegetables.

1. Heat the olive oil in a large, nonstick saucepan over medium heat. Add the onion, carrots, and spice blend. Cook for about 5 minutes or until the onion is translucent.

2. Reduce heat. Add the tomato paste and stir for 1 to 2 minutes.

3. Add the beans and cooked chicken to the pan and stir. Then add the broth and bring to a boil. Reduce the heat and simmer for 30 minutes.

4. Add the spinach to the pot, stir, and then cover.

5. Serve garnished with Parmesan and seasoned to taste with pepper.

**VARIATION TIP:** If you can't find a salt-free Italian spice blend, use ½ teaspoon each of oregano, garlic powder, and sage.

**STORAGE TIP:** Store in the refrigerator in an airtight container for up to 3 days or freeze for up to a month.

. . . . . . . . . . . . . . . . . . . . . . . . . . . . . . . . . . . . . . . .

**Per Serving** Calories: 263; Total fat: 6g; Carbohydrates: 30g; Fiber: 9g; Protein: 25g; Calcium: 114mg; Sodium: 116mg; Potassium: 982mg; Vitamin D: 0mcg; Iron: 5mg; Zinc: 2mg

# Creamy Butternut Squash Soup

✔ ONE-POT

**SERVES 2**

**PREP TIME:** 10 MINUTES
**COOK TIME:** 15 MINUTES

4 cups low-sodium
chicken broth

1 (15-ounce) can light
coconut milk

2 teaspoons olive oil

1 tablespoon chili paste

½ teaspoon ground cumin

¼ teaspoon ground ginger

¼ teaspoon
ground coriander

1 (10-ounce) bag frozen
butternut squash

Nonfat Greek yogurt, for
garnish (optional)

This comforting soup is smooth, delicious, and loaded with beta-carotene. It's a nice way to fit a serving of vegetables into your meal plan. The coconut milk gives it a satisfying, rich flavor and a sweet flair. You can use a regular blender if you don't have an immersion blender, or you can cook the squash separately and then purée it before adding it to the soup.

1. In a medium bowl, whisk together the chicken broth and coconut milk until well combined and set aside.

2. Heat the olive oil over low to medium heat in a large Dutch oven or stockpot. Add the chili paste, cumin, ginger, and coriander and stir for 1 minute.

3. Whisk in the broth and coconut milk mixture. Add the squash, stir, and bring the soup to a boil, then reduce the heat to low.

4. Simmer for 14 minutes, stirring occasionally, or until the squash is tender.

5. Remove the soup from the heat and, using an immersion blender or food processor, blend the soup until it is creamy.

6. Serve garnished with a dollop of yogurt (if using).

**SUBSTITUTION TIP:** You can substitute ¼ teaspoon of cayenne pepper for the chili paste, or if you prefer less spice, 2 teaspoons of tomato paste.

**Per Serving** Calories: 630; Total fat: 54g; Carbohydrates: 35g; Fiber: 3g; Protein: 17g; Calcium: 117mg; Sodium: 290mg; Potassium: 1173mg; Vitamin D: 0mcg; Iron: 10mg; Zinc: 2mg

# Stuffed Pepper Soup

✓ ONE-POT

**SERVES 3**

**PREP TIME:** 15 MINUTES
**COOK TIME:** 1 HOUR,
10 MINUTES

3 cups water

1 cup brown rice

2 teaspoons olive oil

¾ pound 90 percent lean
ground beef

2 large green bell
peppers, diced

¼ cup finely chopped
sweet onion

2 tablespoons
tomato paste

4 cups low-sodium
beef broth

1 (15-ounce) can
low-sodium
diced tomatoes

1 teaspoon dried oregano

Stuffed bell peppers are a staple comfort food in many households; who knew that those familiar delicious flavors could be a hearty soup as well? Made with lean beef and bursting with peppers, tomatoes, and fiber-rich brown rice, this meal is ideal to settle down with after a long day.

1. Bring the water to a boil in a large saucepan over high heat. Add the rice and cook according to package directions, about 45 minutes. Set aside.

2. While the rice is cooking, heat the oil in a Dutch oven over medium heat, then add the ground beef and cook until completely browned, about 8 minutes. Drain the fat and set the Dutch oven back on the heat.

3. Add the peppers and onion and sauté for 5 minutes until tender. Stir in the tomato paste and cook for 1 more minute.

4. Add the broth, tomatoes, and oregano along with the cooked rice, and bring the soup to a boil. Reduce the heat to low, simmer for 30 minutes, and serve.

**SUBSTITUTION TIP:** You can substitute ground lean turkey breast for the beef. You can also swap a cup of cooked barley for the rice or use quick-cooking brown rice to save a little time.

**STORAGE TIP:** Store in the refrigerator in an airtight container for up to 3 days or freeze for up to a month.

. . . . . . . . . . . . . . . . . . . . . . . . . . . . . . . . . . . . . . . . . . . . . . . . . . .

**Per Serving** Calories: 518; Total fat: 17g; Carbohydrates: 62g; Fiber: 7g; Protein: 30g; Calcium: 72mg; Sodium: 95mg; Potassium: 1193mg; Vitamin D: 0mcg; Iron: 5mg; Zinc: 7mg

# Hearty Black Bean Chili

✔ **MAKE-AHEAD**
✔ **ONE-POT**
✔ **VEGETARIAN**

**SERVES 2 TO 3**

**PREP TIME:** 10 MINUTES
**COOK TIME:** 35 MINUTES

2 teaspoons olive oil

1 large green bell
  pepper, diced

½ cup finely chopped
  sweet onion

1 (15-ounce) can no-salt-
  added diced tomatoes and
  green chiles

1 (15-ounce) can black
  beans, drained and rinsed

1 cup frozen corn

1 (8-ounce) can
  tomato sauce

2 tablespoons chili powder

1 teaspoon ground cumin

Nonfat Greek yogurt,
  for garnish

¼ cup shredded sharp
  cheddar cheese,
  for garnish

Canned vegetables bring this dish together very quickly, making it a superb choice for convenient meal prep menus. It also freezes well. You can store it in the refrigerator for up to 3 days or in the freezer for up to 3 months. Want to make this dish vegan? No problem! Simply omit the yogurt and cheese garnish or substitute with your favorite vegan yogurt or cheese.

1. Heat the oil in a medium stockpot over medium heat and sauté the pepper and onion until softened, about 5 minutes.

2. Add the tomatoes, beans, corn, tomato sauce, chili powder, and cumin. Stir to combine and bring to a boil. Reduce the heat to low and simmer for 30 minutes.

3. Ladle the chili into 2 bowls, garnish each bowl with a dollop of yogurt and 2 tablespoons of shredded cheese, and serve.

**SUBSTITUTION TIP:** You can use pinto beans or a mixture of pinto and black beans.

**INGREDIENT TIP:** Stock up on no-salt-added tomatoes. If you can't find the no-salt type, look for reduced sodium.

. . . . . . . . . . . . . . . . . . . . . . . . . . . . . . . . . . . . . . . . .

**Per Serving** Calories: 477; Total fat: 13g; Carbohydrates: 76g; Fiber: 24g; Protein: 24g; Calcium: 289mg; Sodium: 371mg; Potassium: 1651mg; Vitamin D: 0mcg; Iron: 8mg; Zinc: 4mg

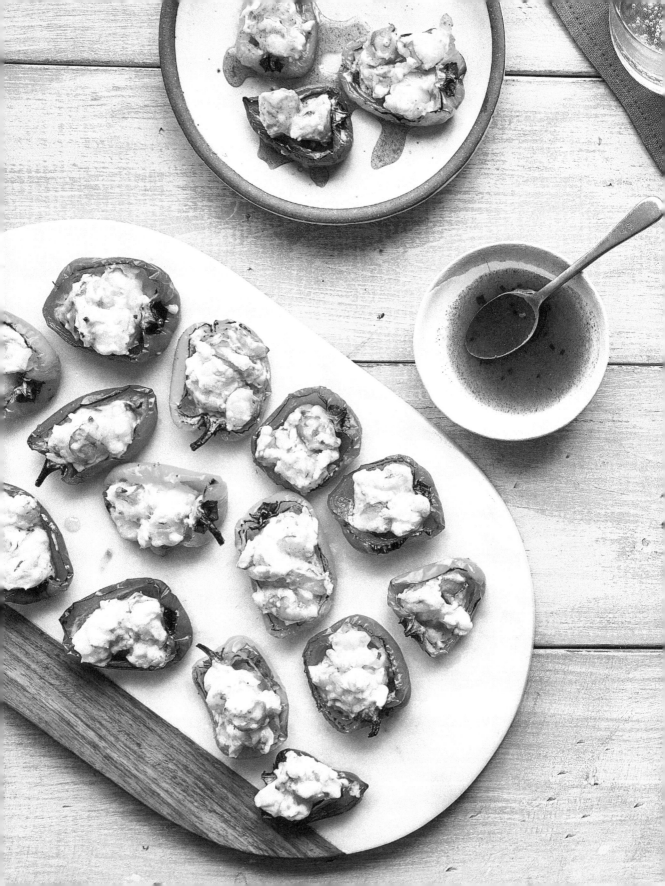

# 4
# SNACKS

# Protein-Powered Iced Coffee

✔ 30 MINUTES OR LESS
✔ ONE-POT
✔ VEGETARIAN

**SERVES 2**

**PREP TIME:** 5 MINUTES

2½ cups black
 coffee, cooled

1 cup 1 percent milk

1 scoop vanilla
 protein powder

1 teaspoon
 ground cinnamon

6 ice cubes

Store-bought iced coffee is undeniably delicious but never look up how many calories, saturated fat, and sugar these frothy beverages contain. It is lucky this shaken-not-stirred homemade creation is nutritious and has all the satisfying lusciousness of its counterpart. The vanilla powder adds protein, and the cinnamon gives it a little sweetness. Fill your to-go cup or enjoy this for the afternoon slump to help you power through the rest of the day.

1. Pour the coffee and milk into a blender. Add the protein powder, cinnamon, and ice.

2. Blend until smooth, pour into two glasses, and serve immediately.

**VARIATION TIP:** Add a whipped coffee (dalgona-style) topping! Mix 2 tablespoons instant decaf coffee, 2 tablespoons granulated sugar, and 2 tablespoons boiling water. Using a hand mixer, beat until it becomes a light caramel color with stiff peaks. Top each iced coffee with this creamy mixture.

. . . . . . . . . . . . . . . . . . . . . . . . . . . . . . . . . . . . . . . . . . . . . . . .

**Per Serving** Calories: 106; Total fat: 1g; Carbohydrates: 11g; Fiber: 1g; Protein: 13g; Calcium: 266mg; Sodium: 107mg; Potassium: 314mg; Vitamin D: 1mcg; Iron: 0mg; Zinc: 2mg

# Berry Crunch Yogurt Parfait

✓ **30 MINUTES OR LESS**
✓ **ONE-POT**
✓ **VEGETARIAN**

**SERVES 2**

**PREP TIME:** 5 MINUTES

½ cup blueberries

¼ cup raspberries

2 cups plain low-fat or nonfat Greek yogurt, divided

¼ cup granola with nuts and seeds, divided

This parfait is something I could eat every day. The beauty of this pleasing treat is its simplicity; it can be whipped up in less than five minutes. You can switch out the berries for other fruit you happen to have in your refrigerator. It's the perfect DASH snack!

*1.* In a small bowl, toss together the blueberries and raspberries.

*2.* Spoon ⅓ cup of yogurt into a tall glass or parfait dish. Top with 1 tablespoon of the granola. Add 2 tablespoons of the mixed berries.

*3.* Repeat the layers two more times, ending with berries on top.

*4.* Repeat with the second glass and serve.

**SUBSTITUTION TIP:** You can also use frozen berries or strawberries here, but make sure to defrost them first. Adding slices of bananas also gives this parfait a sweeter kick.

. . . . . . . . . . . . . . . . . . . . . . . . . . . . . . . . . . . . . . . . . . .

**Per Serving** Calories: 236; Total fat: 5g; Carbohydrates: 34g; Fiber: 3g; Protein: 15g; Calcium: 467mg; Sodium: 179mg; Potassium: 689mg; Vitamin D: 0mcg; Iron: 1mg; Zinc: 3mg

# Spiced Roasted Chickpeas

**SERVES 4**

**PREP TIME:** 5 MINUTES
**COOK TIME:** 25 MINUTES

1 (15-ounce) can chickpeas, drained and rinsed

1 tablespoon olive or avocado oil

1 teaspoon garlic powder

1 teaspoon paprika

¼ teaspoon salt

Chickpeas, also called garbanzo beans, are high in protein, fiber, folate, and iron. They contain a plant sterol called sitosterol, which has been shown to help lower blood cholesterol levels. And the best part? You can turn this humble legume into a crunchy and satisfying snack in half an hour.

1. Preheat the oven to 400°F. Line a baking sheet with parchment paper or a silicone mat.

2. Spread the chickpeas on the baking sheet and drizzle with oil.

3. In a small bowl, mix the garlic powder, paprika, and salt. Sprinkle the mixture over the chickpeas and toss to coat.

4. Roast the chickpeas for 20 to 25 minutes, until crisp and lightly browned.

5. Remove the chickpeas from the baking sheet and enjoy them immediately.

**SUBSTITUTION TIP:** For a sweeter flavor, substitute cinnamon and nutmeg for the garlic powder and paprika.

**STORAGE TIP:** You can store these in an airtight container for up to 3 days, but they may soften.

. . . . . . . . . . . . . . . . . . . . . . . . . . . . . . . . . . . . . . . . . . . . . . . . . . .

**Per Serving** Calories: 136; Total fat: 5g; Carbohydrates: 17g; Fiber: 5g; Protein: 6g; Calcium: 32mg; Sodium: 151mg; Potassium: 201mg; Vitamin D: 0mcg; Iron: 2mg; Zinc: 1mg

# Lemony Bean Dip with Pita Triangles

✓ **30 MINUTES OR LESS**
✓ **ONE-POT**
✓ **VEGETARIAN**

**SERVES 2 TO 3**

**PREP TIME:** 15 MINUTES
**COOK TIME:** 10 MINUTES

3 whole-wheat pita pock-
ets, cut into eighths

Nonstick cooking spray

1 (15-ounce) can cannellini
beans, drained

1 garlic clove

2 tablespoons
crumbled feta

2 teaspoons avocado oil

1 lemon

1 tablespoon chopped
parsley, for garnish

This dip is like having two fabulous snacks: the velvety bean purée and the crunchy golden pita chips. Delicious! They're loaded with fiber, vitamins A and C, and protein. You can make this dip ahead, as it stores well. In addition to the pita chips, you can also serve it with carrot sticks, celery, bell peppers, cucumbers, or any other vegetable of your choosing.

1. Preheat the oven to 400°F.

2. Arrange the pita pieces on the baking sheet and spray them on both sides with cooking spray. Bake for 10 minutes until lightly toasted. Remove from the oven and set aside.

3. Add the beans, garlic, feta, and oil to a food processor. Grate some lemon zest from the whole lemon into the processor (about ¼ teaspoon). Cut the lemon in half and squeeze in the juice from one half. Cut the remaining lemon half into two quarters. Reserving a quarter for garnish, squeeze the rest of the lemon juice into the processor.

4. Pulse until the mixture is smooth.

5. Transfer the dip to a small bowl, garnish with the lemon wedge and parsley, and serve with the pita chips.

**STORAGE TIP:** This dip can be stored in an airtight container in the refrigerator for up to 5 days.

. . . . . . . . . . . . . . . . . . . . . . . . . . . . . . . . . . . . . . . . . . . . . . . . .

**Per Serving** Calories: 354; Total fat: 8g; Carbohydrates: 56g; Fiber: 12g; Protein: 17g; Calcium: 106mg; Sodium: 267mg; Potassium: 656mg; Vitamin D: 0mcg; Iron: 4mg; Zinc: 2mg

# Crostini with Ricotta & Fig Jam

✔ 30 MINUTES OR LESS
✔ ONE-POT
✔ VEGETARIAN

**SERVES 2**

**PREP TIME:** 15 MINUTES
**COOK TIME:** 5 MINUTES

10 (¼-inch) baguette slices

½ cup part-skim
  ricotta cheese

¼ teaspoon cinnamon

1 tablespoon fig jam, or
  other fruit preserve

¼ cup chopped walnuts

¼ cup chopped apple

These not only taste delicious but also look beautiful on a small platter. You can mix up the flavors with different jams or garnish toppings and easily double the recipe for company. Fig jam can be found with the condiments or nut butters or with the jams and jellies. In a pinch, you can substitute honey or apricot jam. The ricotta provides some DASH-friendly dairy, and the toppings add extra vitamins and potassium.

1. Lightly toast the baguette slices in a toaster oven or on a baking sheet in an oven preheated to 300°F, for 3 to 5 minutes.

2. In a small bowl, mix the ricotta with the cinnamon. Top each toast with a little less than a tablespoon of this mixture.

3. Top evenly with the jam, nuts, and apple and serve.

**SUBSTITUTION TIP:** Substitute chopped peaches or chopped prunes for the apples. You can also use canned peaches or pears. Look for canned fruit packed in juice or water and drain it well.

. . . . . . . . . . . . . . . . . . . . . . . . . . . . . . . . . . . . . . . . . . . . .

**Per Serving** Calories: 435; Total fat: 16g; Carbohydrates: 56g; Fiber: 3g; Protein: 18g; Calcium: 231mg; Sodium: 521mg; Potassium: 260mg; Vitamin D: 0mcg; Iron: 4mg; Zinc: 2mg

# Seedy Granola Squares

✓ ONE-POT

✓ VEGETARIAN

**MAKES 6 SQUARES**

**PREP TIME:** 15 MINUTES

**COOK TIME:** 20 MINUTES

Nonstick cooking spray

½ cup whole-wheat flour

½ cup oats

¾ teaspoon baking powder

⅛ teaspoon salt

⅔ cup packed brown sugar

3 tablespoons unsalted butter, softened

1 large egg

¼ teaspoon pure vanilla extract

½ cup granola

¼ cup sunflower seed kernels

Seeds such as sunflower, poppy, sesame, chia, and flax are all filled with healthy fats. They are calorie-dense due to this fat content, so a little goes a long way. Adding seeds to recipes like these healthy bars is a delicious way to include them in your diet. Try roasted pumpkin seeds in place of the sunflower seeds for a burst of flavor.

1. Preheat the oven to 350°F. Coat a 9-by-5-inch loaf pan with cooking spray or line it with parchment paper.

2. In a small bowl, combine the flour, oats, baking powder, and salt. Set aside.

3. With an electric or hand mixer in a large bowl, cream the sugar and butter until the mixture is smooth and pale.

4. Add the egg and vanilla and beat well, scraping down the sides of the bowl. Stir in the flour mixture, granola, and seeds. Transfer the mixture to the prepared loaf pan.

5. Bake for 20 minutes or until lightly browned. Allow the loaf to cool 10 minutes, then cut into 2-by-3-inch squares.

**VARIATION TIP:** You can add in 3 tablespoons of dried fruit, or you can change the butter to vegetable oil. However, butter adds rich flavor to these squares, and in this small amount, it doesn't break any DASH rules.

**STORAGE TIP:** Store in an airtight container for up to a week.

. . . . . . . . . . . . . . . . . . . . . . . . . . . . . . . . . . . . . . . . . . . . .

**Per Serving (1 square)** Calories: 330; Total fat: 13g; Carbohydrates: 48g; Fiber: 3g; Protein: 7g; Calcium: 75mg; Sodium: 75mg; Potassium: 270mg; Vitamin D: 0mcg; Iron: 2mg; Zinc: 1mg

# Peanut-Powered Snack Bars

✔ VEGETARIAN

**MAKES 6 BARS**

**PREP TIME:** 15 MINUTES
**COOK TIME:** 10 MINUTES

⅔ cup peanut
 butter powder

⅓ cup water

1 egg white, beaten

1 tablespoon avocado oil

1 cup quick oats

3 tablespoons honey

1 teaspoon pure
 vanilla extract

⅛ teaspoon salt

1 tablespoon mini semi-
 sweet chocolate chips

These peanut butter and chocolate treats can help you when the candy-bar craving strikes. They are also perfect as a midday snack to hold you over until dinner. If you don't have peanut butter powder, you can use two-thirds of a cup of peanut or almond butter instead. The peanut butter powder brand I like is Crazy Richard's.

1. Preheat the oven to 350°F. Line a 9-by-5-inch loaf pan with parchment paper.

2. In a medium bowl, mix the peanut butter powder and water until smooth. Beat in the egg white and oil.

3. Add the oats, honey, vanilla, and salt and mix well. Then fold in the chocolate chips.

4. Spoon the mixture into the pan and press it into an even layer.

5. Bake the mixture for 10 minutes. Remove the pan from the oven and let it cool.

6. Remove the baked snack from the pan and cut it evenly into 6 small bars.

**STORAGE TIP:** Store the bars at room temperature in an airtight container, separated with wax paper, or freeze them for up to 2 months.

. . . . . . . . . . . . . . . . . . . . . . . . . . . . . . . . . . . . . . . . . . . . . . . .

**Per Serving (1 bar)** Calories: 255; Total fat: 12g; Carbohydrates: 31g; Fiber: 4g; Protein: 8g; Calcium: 23mg; Sodium: 64mg; Potassium: 206mg; Vitamin D: 0mcg; Iron: 2mg; Zinc: 1mg

# Mixed Berry Muffins

✔ 30 MINUTES OR LESS
✔ VEGETARIAN

**MAKES 6 MUFFINS**

**PREP TIME:** 10 MINUTES
**COOK TIME:** 18 MINUTES

Nonstick cooking spray

½ cup unbleached
 all-purpose flour

½ cup oats

3 tablespoons packed
 brown sugar

1 teaspoon baking powder

⅛ teaspoon salt

½ cup milk

1 large egg

2 tablespoons avocado oil

½ teaspoon pure
 vanilla extract

½ cup blueberries

½ cup raspberries

Is it my imagination, or are store-bought muffins getting bigger? Sometimes you almost need two hands to hold one of these monstrous sugar- and fat-packed creations. However, homemade muffins like the ones this recipe makes are smaller, and these are also lower in sugar and higher in fiber. Whip up a batch when you are craving a sweet, satisfying treat.

1. Preheat the oven to 350°F. Spray a 6-cup muffin tin with nonstick cooking spray.

2. In a medium bowl, whisk together the flour, oats, sugar, baking powder, and salt until well combined.

3. In a measuring cup, stir together the milk, egg, oil, and vanilla until blended. Add the wet ingredients to the dry ingredients and stir until just combined.

4. Gently fold in the berries, carefully so as not to over-work the batter. Spoon the batter into the muffin cups, filling them two-thirds full.

5. Bake the muffins for 15 to 18 minutes or until lightly browned. Let the muffins cool, then remove them from the pan and serve.

**STORAGE TIP:** Store the muffins in an airtight container for up to 3 days in the refrigerator or freeze them in a sealed freezer bag for up to 3 months.

. . . . . . . . . . . . . . . . . . . . . . . . . . . . . . . . . . . . . . . . . . . . . . . . . . .

**Per Serving (1 muffin)** Calories: 186; Total fat: 7g; Carbohydrates: 25g; Fiber: 3g; Protein: 5g; Calcium: 79mg; Sodium: 75mg; Potassium: 221mg; Vitamin D: 0mcg; Iron: 1mg; Zinc: 1mg

# Whole-Wheat Cranberry Muffins

✔ **30 MINUTES OR LESS**
✔ **ONE-POT**
✔ **VEGETARIAN**

**MAKES 6 MUFFINS**

**PREP TIME:** 10 MINUTES
**COOK TIME:** 18 MINUTES

Nonstick cooking spray

1 cup whole-wheat flour

3 tablespoons packed
 brown sugar

1 teaspoon baking powder

⅛ teaspoon salt

½ cup milk

1 large egg

2 tablespoons avocado oil

½ teaspoon pure
 maple extract

¼ cup dried cranberries

¼ cup plain
 walnuts, chopped

These crunchy, fiber-packed muffins make an excellent DASH snack to enjoy midmorning or midday with a glass of milk. The hint of maple paired with tart cranberries is a pleasing sweet-and-sour taste experience. To boost nutrition, you can add a wide variety of fruits, including dried cherries or apricots. To pack in more protein and healthy fat, add more nuts or seeds.

1. Heat the oven to 350°F. Spray a 6-cup muffin tin with nonstick cooking spray.

2. In a medium bowl, whisk the flour, sugar, baking powder, and salt until well combined.

3. In a measuring cup, stir together the milk, egg, oil, and maple extract until blended. Add the wet ingredients to the dry ingredients and stir until just combined.

4. Stir in the cranberries and nuts. Spoon the batter into the muffin cups, filling them two-thirds full.

5. Bake the muffins for 15 to 18 minutes until lightly browned. Cool for 10 minutes, then serve.

**STORAGE TIP:** Store the muffins in an airtight bag or container for up to 3 days in the refrigerator or freeze them for up to 3 months.

. . . . . . . . . . . . . . . . . . . . . . . . . . . . . . . . . . . . . . . . . . . . .

**Per Serving (1 muffin)** Calories: 201; Total fat: 10g; Carbohydrates: 25g; Fiber: 3g; Protein: 5g; Calcium: 80mg; Sodium: 75mg; Potassium: 226mg; Vitamin D: 0mcg; Iron: 1mg; Zinc: 1mg

# Grilled Shrimp-Stuffed Poppers

✔ **30 MINUTES OR LESS**
✔ **ONE-POT**

**SERVES 2**

**PREP TIME:** 15 MINUTES
**COOK TIME:** 10 MINUTES

8 mini sweet bell peppers, halved and seeded

4 ounces light Neufchatel cheese (or low-fat cream cheese or goat cheese), softened

1 cup cooked shrimp, diced

½ teaspoon paprika

1 teaspoon hot chili sauce

1 teaspoon honey

If you enjoy jalapeño poppers, you'll love this healthier version. They still have all of the traditional popper flavors you love, but with less fat and fewer calories. By skipping the breading, using light cream cheese, and grilling them, you eliminate all the aspects of the classic dish that are less healthy without sacrificing delicious flavor. No grill? No problem. See the tip for making these in the oven.

1. Heat a grill to medium-high, or around 400°F. Line a baking sheet with parchment paper.

2. Place the peppers on the baking sheet.

3. In a small bowl, mix together the Neufchatel cheese, shrimp, and paprika until well combined.

4. Stuff each pepper with a spoonful of the cream cheese mixture and place them on a grill pan.

5. Grill for 10 minutes, until the peppers are tender and the cheese is warm. Transfer the peppers to a medium plate.

6. Evenly drizzle the peppers with the chili sauce and honey and serve.

**COOKING TIP:** If you don't have a grill, you can bake these in a 425°F oven for 15 to 20 minutes.

......................................................................

**Per Serving** Calories: 286; Total fat: 14g; Carbohydrates: 30g; Fiber: 4g; Protein: 14g; Calcium: 129mg; Sodium: 412mg; Potassium: 937mg; Vitamin D: 0mcg; Iron: 2mg; Zinc: 1mg

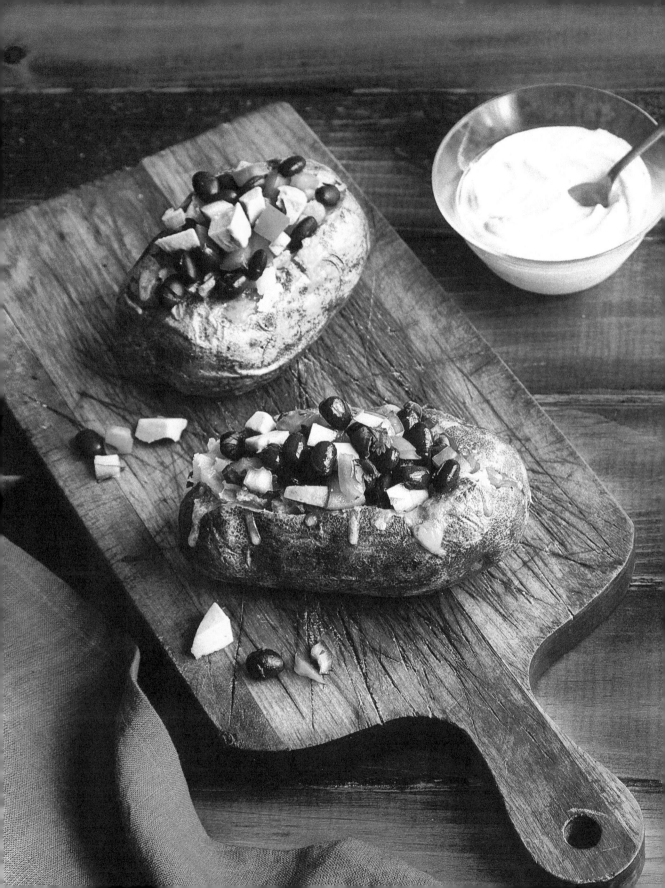

# 5
# MEATLESS MAINS

# Moroccan-Inspired Tagine with Chickpeas & Vegetables

✓ ONE-POT
✓ VEGAN

**SERVES 2 TO 3**

**PREP TIME:** 10 MINUTES
**COOK TIME:** 45 MINUTES

2 teaspoons olive oil

1 cup chopped carrots

½ cup finely chopped onion

1 sweet potato, diced

1 cup low-sodium
   vegetable broth

¼ teaspoon
   ground cinnamon

⅛ teaspoon salt

1½ cups chopped bell
   peppers, any color

3 ripe plum tomatoes,
   seeded and finely chopped

1 tablespoon tomato paste

1 garlic clove, pressed
   or minced

1 (15-ounce) can chickpeas,
   drained and rinsed

½ cup chopped
   dried apricots

1 teaspoon curry powder

½ teaspoon paprika

½ teaspoon turmeric

A tagine is a traditional piece of Moroccan cookware with a cone-shaped lid that traps all the rising steam and condenses it back into the dish. You don't have to use a tagine for cooking this North African-inspired stew; any vessel with a lid will do, such as the Dutch oven or saucepan used in this recipe. The cinnamon and spice mix in this nutrient-packed dish give it its unique flavor profile. To complete the meal, serve over couscous.

1. Heat the oil over medium heat in a large Dutch oven or saucepan. Add the carrots and onion and cook until the onion is translucent, about 4 minutes.

2. Add the sweet potato, broth, cinnamon, and salt and cook for 5 to 6 minutes, until the broth is slightly reduced.

3. Add the peppers, tomatoes, tomato paste, and garlic. Stir and cook for another 5 minutes.

4. Add the chickpeas, apricots, curry powder, paprika, and turmeric to the pot. Bring all to a boil, then reduce the heat to low, cover, simmer for about 30 minutes, and serve.

**SUBSTITUTION TIP:** You can substitute raisins or dates for the apricots. If you'd like it spicier, add ¼ teaspoon cayenne pepper.

**STORAGE TIP:** Store leftovers in an airtight container in the refrigerator for up to 3 days.

. . . . . . . . . . . . . . . . . . . . . . . . . . . . . . . . . . . . . . . . . . . .

**Per Serving**  Calories: 469; Total fat: 9g; Carbohydrates: 88g; Fiber: 20g; Protein: 16g; Calcium: 156mg; Sodium: 256mg; Potassium: 1587mg; Vitamin D: 0mcg; Iron: 7mg; Zinc: 3mg

# Spaghetti Squash with Maple Glaze & Tofu Crumbles

✓ **VEGETARIAN**

**SERVES 2 TO 3**

**PREP TIME:** 20 MINUTES
**COOK TIME:** 22 MINUTES

2 ounces firm tofu, well-drained

1 small spaghetti squash, halved lengthwise

2½ teaspoons olive oil, divided

⅛ teaspoon salt

½ cup chopped onion

1 teaspoon dried rosemary

¼ cup dry white wine

2 tablespoons maple syrup

½ teaspoon garlic powder

¼ cup shredded Gruyère cheese

Spaghetti squash is one of the surprise ingredients that can be swapped effectively for another one, in this case, "pasta." When you cook this unassuming vegetable, the flesh can be separated into long golden strands resembling, of course, spaghetti. Tofu serves as your protein, completing the meal. The drizzle of garlic-infused maple elevates the dish to fine-dining quality.

1. Put the tofu in a large mesh colander and place over a large bowl to drain.

2. Use a paring knife to score the squash so the steam can vent while it cooks.

3. Place the squash in a medium microwave-safe dish and microwave on high for 5 minutes. Remove the squash from the microwave and allow it to cool.

4. Cut the cooled squash in half on a cutting board. Scoop out the seeds, then place the squash havles into a 9-by-11-inch baking dish. Drizzle the squash with half a teaspoon of olive oil and season it with the salt, then cover it with wax paper and put it back in the microwave for 5 more minutes on high, or until the skin is easily pierced with a fork. Once it's cooked, scrape the squash strands with a fork into a small bowl and cover it to keep it warm.

5. While the squash is cooking, heat 1 teaspoon of oil in a large skillet over medium-high heat. Add the onion and sauté for 5 minutes. Add the rosemary and stir for 1 minute, until fragrant.

CONTINUED ▶

6. In the same skillet, add the remaining oil. Crumble the tofu into the skillet and stir fry until lightly browned, about 4 minutes, and transfer it to a small bowl.

7. Add the wine, maple syrup, and garlic powder to the skillet and stir to combine. Cook for 2 minutes until slightly reduced and thickened. Remove from the heat.

8. Evenly divide the squash between two plates, then top it with the tofu mixture. Drizzle the maple glaze over the top, then add the grated cheese.

VARIATION TIP: You can skip the cheese or use vegan cheese to make this dish vegan.

Per Serving  Calories: 330; Total fat: 15g; Carbohydrates: 36g; Fiber: 5g; Protein: 12g; Calcium: 457mg; Sodium: 326mg; Potassium: 474mg; Vitamin D: 0mcg; Iron: 2mg; Zinc: 2mg

# Stuffed Tex-Mex Baked Potatoes

✔ ONE-POT

✔ VEGETARIAN

**SERVES 2**

**PREP TIME:** 10 MINUTES
**COOK TIME:** 45 MINUTES

2 large Idaho potatoes

½ cup black beans, rinsed and drained

¼ cup store-bought salsa

1 avocado, diced

1 teaspoon freshly squeezed lime juice

½ cup nonfat plain Greek yogurt

¼ teaspoon reduced-sodium taco seasoning

¼ cup shredded sharp cheddar cheese

Potatoes are an excellent source of fiber, Vitamin C, and potassium. They are also a perfect DASH canvas on which to add other nutrient-dense foods. These potatoes are also a great lunch idea the day after you make the Hearty Black Bean Chili (page 51). Just substitute the chili for the salsa and beans. You can also use leftover cooked chicken or lentils if you'd like more protein.

1. Preheat the oven to 400°F.

2. Scrub the potatoes. Using a paring knife, cut an "X" into the top of each. Place the potatoes directly on the oven rack and bake for 45 minutes until they are tender.

3. In a small bowl, stir together the beans and salsa and set aside. In another small bowl, mix together the avocado and lime juice and set aside. In a third small bowl, stir together the yogurt and the taco seasoning until well blended.

4. When the potatoes are baked, carefully open them up. Top each potato with the bean and salsa mixture, avocado, seasoned yogurt, and cheddar cheese, evenly dividing each component, and serve.

**INGREDIENT TIP:** Fresh salsa from the deli section is often lower in sodium than jarred salsas.

. . . . . . . . . . . . . . . . . . . . . . . . . . . . . . . . . . . . . . . . . . . . . . . . . . . . .

**Per Serving** Calories: 624; Total fat: 21g; Carbohydrates: 91g; Fiber:21 g; Protein: 24g; Calcium: 238mg; Sodium: 366mg; Potassium: 2134mg; Vitamin D: 0mcg; Iron: 4mg; Zinc: 3mg

# Lentil-Stuffed Zucchini Boats

✔ MAKE-AHEAD

✔ VEGETARIAN

**SERVES 2**

**PREP TIME:** 35 MINUTES
**COOK TIME:** 45 MINUTES

2 medium zucchini, halved
  lengthwise and seeded

2¼ cups water, divided

1 cup dried green or red
  lentils, rinsed

2 teaspoons olive oil

⅓ cup diced onion

2 tablespoons
  tomato paste

½ teaspoon oregano

¼ teaspoon garlic powder

Pinch salt

¼ cup grated part-skim
  mozzarella cheese

This filling dish substitutes lentils for ground meat, increasing the fiber and reducing the fat, but still providing you with a lovely texture and taste. These zucchini boats are a perfect light dish with no leftovers, but you can double the filling to save time on a future dish. Try it in the Lentil Quinoa Gratin with Butternut Squash (page 74).

1. Preheat the oven to 375°F. Line a baking sheet with parchment paper. Place the zucchini, hollow sides up, on the baking sheet and set aside.

2. In a medium saucepan, bring 2 cups of water to a boil over high heat and add the lentils. Reduce the heat to low, cover, and simmer for 20 to 25 minutes. Drain and set aside.

3. Heat the olive oil in a medium skillet over medium-low heat. Sauté the onions until they are translucent, about 4 minutes. Reduce the heat to low and add the cooked lentils, tomato paste, oregano, garlic powder, and salt. Add the last quarter cup of water and simmer for 3 minutes, until the liquid reduces and forms a sauce. Remove from heat.

4. Stuff each zucchini half with the lentil mixture, dividing it evenly, top with cheese, bake for 25 minutes, and serve. The zucchini should be fork-tender, and the cheese should be melted.

**SUBSTITUTION TIP:** You can skip the cheese or use vegan cheese to make this dish vegan. You can also use ½ cup chopped walnuts in place of half of the lentils.

. . . . . . . . . . . . . . . . . . . . . . . . . . . . . . . . . . . . . . . . . . .

**Per Serving** Calories: 479; Total fat: 9g; Carbohydrates: 74g; Fiber: 14g; Protein: 31g; Calcium: 183mg; Sodium: 206mg; Potassium: 1389mg; Vitamin D: 0mcg; Iron: 8mg; Zinc: 4mg

# Baked Eggplant Parmesan

✔ MAKE-AHEAD
✔ VEGETARIAN

**SERVES 3 TO 4**

**PREP TIME:** 15 MINUTES
**COOK TIME:** 35 MINUTES

1 small to medium eggplant, cut into ¼-inch slices

½ teaspoon salt-free Italian seasoning blend

1 tablespoon olive oil

¼ cup diced onion

½ cup diced yellow or red bell pepper

2 garlic cloves, pressed or minced

1 (8-ounce) can tomato sauce

3 ounces fresh mozzarella, cut into 6 pieces

1 tablespoon grated Parmesan cheese, divided

5 to 6 fresh basil leaves, chopped

This delectable dish has all of the flavors of classic eggplant Parmesan, but with much less fat and fewer calories. Eggplant is a staple vegetarian ingredient because it adds meaty texture to a dish and soaks up the flavors of all the other ingredients. The air fryer cuts down on time and gives the eggplant a nice crispness. If you don't have an air fryer, however, these can be made in a conventional oven. (See tip.)

1. Preheat an oven-style air fryer to 400°F.

2. Working in two batches, place the eggplant slices onto the air-fryer tray, and sprinkle them with Italian seasoning. Bake for 7 minutes. Repeat with the remaining slices, then set them aside on a plate.

3. In a medium skillet, heat the oil over medium heat and sauté the onion and peppers until softened, about 5 minutes. Add the garlic and sauté for 1 to 2 more minutes. Add the tomato sauce and stir to combine. Remove the sauce from the heat.

4. Spray a 9-by-6-inch casserole dish with cooking spray. Spread one-third of the sauce into the bottom of the dish. Layer eggplant slices onto the sauce. Sprinkle with half of the Parmesan cheese. Continue layering the sauce and eggplant, ending with the sauce. Place the mozzarella pieces on the top. Sprinkle the remaining Parmesan evenly over the entire dish.

5. Bake in the oven for 20 minutes. Garnish with fresh basil, cut into four servings, and serve.

**CONTINUED** ▶

## Baked Eggplant Parmesan CONTINUED

**COOKING TIP:** If you don't have an air fryer, place the sliced eggplant onto a large oil-coated baking sheet. Spray the slices with cooking spray and bake for 30 minutes at 400°F.

**STORAGE TIP:** Store leftovers in the refrigerator for up to 3 days.

. . . . . . . . . . . . . . . . . . . . . . . . . . . . . . . . . . . . . . . . . . . . . . . . .

**Per Serving** Calories: 213; Total fat: 12g; Carbohydrates: 20g; Fiber: 7g; Protein: 10g; Calcium: 196mg; Sodium: 222mg; Potassium: 763mg; Vitamin D: 0mcg; Iron: 2mg; Zinc: 1mg

# Summer Barley Pilaf with Yogurt Dill Sauce

**SERVES 2 TO 3**

**PREP TIME:** 15 MINUTES
**COOK TIME:** 30 MINUTES

2⅔ cups low-sodium
  vegetable broth

2 teaspoons avocado oil

1 small zucchini, diced

⅓ cup slivered almonds

2 scallions, sliced, white
  and green parts separated

1 cup barley

½ cup plain nonfat
  Greek yogurt

2 teaspoons grated
  lemon zest

¼ teaspoon dried dill

This dish can be enjoyed year-round, but it's ideal for a summer picnic and can be easily doubled. Barley has a chewier texture than rice. Its fiber content can help reduce blood cholesterol (a risk factor for heart disease). This versatile grain is easy to cook and can be substituted anywhere that you'd use rice.

1. In a large saucepan, bring the broth to a boil.

2. While the broth is coming to a boil, heat the oil in a skillet. Add the zucchini and sauté 3 to 4 minutes. Add the almonds and the white parts of the scallions and sauté for 2 minutes. Remove the mixture from the skillet and transfer it to a small bowl.

3. Add the barley to the skillet and sauté for 2 to 3 minutes to toast. Transfer the barley to the boiling broth and reduce the heat to low, cover, and simmer for 25 minutes or until tender. Remove from the heat and let stand for 10 minutes, or until the liquid is absorbed.

4. While the barley is cooking, in a small bowl stir together the yogurt, lemon zest, and dill and set aside.

5. Fluff the barley with a fork. Add the zucchini, almond, and onion mixture and mix gently.

6. To serve, divide the pilaf between two bowls and drizzle the yogurt over each bowl.

**VARIATION TIP:** If you'd like more protein, you can add cooked chicken to this dish at step 5.

. . . . . . . . . . . . . . . . . . . . . . . . . . . . . . . . . . . . . . . .

**Per Serving** Calories: 545; Total fat: 15g; Carbohydrates: 87g; Fiber: 19g; Protein: 21g; Calcium: 164mg; Sodium: 37mg; Potassium: 694mg; Vitamin D: 0mcg; Iron: 4mg; Zinc: 3mg

# Lentil Quinoa Gratin with Butternut Squash

**SERVES 2 TO 3**

**PREP TIME:** 10 MINUTES
**COOK TIME:** 1 HOUR,
15 MINUTES

### For the Lentils and Squash

Nonstick cooking spray

2 cups water

½ cup dried green or red
lentils, rinsed

Pinch salt

1 teaspoon olive oil, divided

½ cup quinoa

¼ cup diced shallot

2 cups frozen cubed
butternut squash

¼ cup low-fat milk

1 teaspoon chopped
fresh rosemary

Freshly ground black pepper

### For the Gratin Topping

¼ cup panko bread crumbs
or other bread crumbs

1 teaspoon olive oil

⅓ cup shredded
Gruyère cheese

Gratins sound incredibly fattening, but don't worry: The cheesy bread crumb topping here has less saturated fat than a traditional gratin but all the flavor. All the components might seem intimidating, but this superb dish is well worth the time. The lentils add extra fiber to the dish, and the butternut squash is a great source of vitamin A and potassium. Using frozen squash saves time and effort, although you can also use fresh if you have it on hand. (See tip.)

**To Make the Lentils and Squash**

1. Preheat the oven to 400°F. Spray a 1½-quart casserole dish or an 8-by-8-inch baking dish with cooking spray.

2. In a medium saucepan, stir together the water, lentils, and salt and bring to a boil over medium-high heat. Once the water is boiling, reduce the heat to low, cover, and simmer for 20 to 25 minutes. Then drain and transfer the lentils to a large bowl and set aside.

3. In the same saucepan, heat ½ teaspoon of oil over medium heat. Add the quinoa and quickly stir for 1 minute, to toast it lightly. Cook according to the package directions, about 20 minutes.

4. While the quinoa cooks, heat the remaining olive oil in a medium skillet over medium-low heat. Add the shallots and sauté them until they are translucent, about 3 minutes. Add the squash, milk, and rosemary and cook for 1 to 2 minutes. Remove from the heat and transfer to the lentil bowl. Add in the quinoa and gently toss all together.

5. Season with pepper to taste.

6. Transfer the mixture to the casserole dish.

**To Make the Gratin Topping**

7. In a small bowl, mix the panko bread crumbs with the olive oil. Sprinkle the bread crumbs evenly over the casserole and top them with the cheese.

8. Bake the casserole for 25 minutes and serve.

**INGREDIENT TIP:** Fresh squash works well here, too. Cut the squash in half, remove the seeds, and then cook the squash (8 to 12 minutes in the microwave, or 1 hour in a 350°F oven), peel it, and cut it into cubes.

**PREP TIP:** If you batch-cook dried lentils, you can freeze them in quart bags to save time in your recipes.

**STORAGE TIP:** Store the leftovers in the refrigerator for up to 3 days.

. . . . . . . . . . . . . . . . . . . . . . . . . . . . . . . . . . . . . . . . . . . . . . . . .

**Per Serving** Calories: 576; Total fat: 15g; Carbohydrates: 87g; Fiber: 12g; Protein: 28g; Calcium: 351mg; Sodium: 329mg; Potassium: 1176mg; Vitamin D: 0mcg; Iron: 7mg; Zinc: 4mg

# Brown Rice Casserole with Cottage Cheese

✔ BUDGET-SAVER
✔ VEGETARIAN

**SERVES 2 TO 3**

**PREP TIME:** 10 MINUTES
**COOK TIME:** 45 MINUTES

Nonstick cooking spray

1 cup quick-cooking brown rice

1 teaspoon olive oil

½ cup diced sweet onion

1 (10-ounce) bag of fresh spinach

1½ cups low-fat cottage cheese

1 tablespoon grated Parmesan cheese

¼ cup sunflower seed kernels

This meal comes together in a snap thanks to quick-cooking rice and fresh spinach. You will be reminded of a rich, cheesy Florentine-style risotto when you take your first bite. Eat it as a complete meal or as a side dish for four. This tasty casserole is an easy DASH comfort food to put into regular rotation and is also great as leftovers.

1. Preheat the oven to 375°F. Spray a small 1½-quart casserole dish with cooking spray.

2. Cook the rice according to the package directions. Set aside.

3. Heat the oil in a large nonstick skillet over medium-low heat. Add the onion and sauté for 3 to 4 minutes. Add the spinach and cover the skillet, cooking for 1 to 2 minutes until the spinach wilts. Remove the skillet from the heat.

4. In a medium bowl, mix together the rice, spinach mixture, and cottage cheese. Transfer the mixture to the prepared casserole dish. Top with the Parmesan cheese and sunflower seeds, bake for 25 minutes until lightly browned, and serve.

**SUBSTITUTION TIP:** You can use regular brown rice, but it will increase the cooking time by 30 to 40 minutes.

**STORAGE TIP:** Store any leftovers in the refrigerator in an airtight container for 3 days or freeze for up to 3 months.

. . . . . . . . . . . . . . . . . . . . . . . . . . . . . . . . . . . . . . . . .

**Per Serving** Calories: 334; Total fat: 9g; Carbohydrates: 47g; Fiber: 5g; Protein: 19g; Calcium: 185mg; Sodium: 425mg; Potassium: 553mg; Vitamin D: 0mcg; Iron: 3mg; Zinc: 2mg

# Quinoa-Stuffed Peppers

✔ VEGETARIAN

**SERVES 2**

**PREP TIME:** 10 MINUTES
**COOK TIME:** 35 MINUTES

2 large green bell
  peppers, halved

1½ teaspoons olive
  oil, divided

½ cup quinoa

½ cup minced onion

1 garlic clove, pressed
  or minced

1 cup chopped
  portobello mushrooms

3 tablespoons grated
  Parmesan cheese, divided

4 ounces tomato sauce

These are a meatless twist on traditional stuffed peppers, which are usually made with ground beef. Using extra-lean ground beef is DASH-approved, but you won't miss it here, because the quinoa and mushrooms pack in the protein and taste. Try adding a few different wild mushrooms, such as shiitake or oyster, with the portobellos for a different flavor profile.

1. Preheat the oven to 400°F. Line a baking sheet with parchment paper.

2. Place the pepper halves on the baking sheet. Brush the insides of peppers with ½ teaspoon olive oil and bake for 10 minutes. Remove the baking sheet from the oven and set aside.

3. While the peppers bake, cook the quinoa in a large saucepan over medium heat according to the package directions and set aside.

4. Heat the remaining oil in a medium-size skillet over medium heat. Add the onion and sauté until it's translucent, about 3 minutes. Add the garlic and cook for 1 minute. Add the mushrooms to the skillet, reduce the heat to medium-low, cover, and cook for 5 to 6 minutes or until the mushrooms are tender. Uncover, and if there's still liquid in the pan, reduce the heat and cook until the liquid evaporates.

5. Add the mushroom mixture, 1 tablespoon of Parmesan, and the tomato sauce to the quinoa and gently stir to combine.

CONTINUED ▶

6. Carefully spoon the quinoa mixture into each pepper half and sprinkle with the remaining Parmesan. Return the peppers to the oven, bake for 10 to 15 more minutes until tender, and serve.

**INGREDIENT TIP:** For firmer quinoa, toast it in ½ teaspoon of olive oil in the pot for 1 minute before adding the water.

**STORAGE TIP:** Store leftovers in an airtight container in the refrigerator for up to 3 days.

. . . . . . . . . . . . . . . . . . . . . . . . . . . . . . . . . . . . . . . . . . . . . . . . . . . .

**Per Serving** Calories: 292; Total fat: 9g; Carbohydrates: 45g; Fiber: 8g; Protein: 12g; Calcium: 122mg; Sodium: 154mg; Potassium: 929mg; Vitamin D: 0mcg; Iron: 3mg; Zinc: 2mg

# Black Bean Burgers

✓ **BUDGET-SAVER**

✓ **VEGAN**

**MAKES 4 BURGERS**

**PREP TIME:** 15 MINUTES
**COOK TIME:** 20 MINUTES

½ cup quick-cooking
  brown rice

2 teaspoons canola
  oil, divided

½ cup finely
  chopped carrots

¼ cup finely chopped onion

1 (15-ounce) can black
  beans, drained and rinsed

1 tablespoon salt-free
  mesquite seasoning blend

4 small, hard rolls

Burgers are the ultimate get-together meal. Something is charming about adding all the toppings and biting into all the different textures and flavors. The black beans in this meatless burger recipe are high in fiber and a good source of iron and folate. Mesquite flavor seasoning creates a similar taste profile to "regular" burgers, but feel free to change up the seasoning. Give your burgers a bigger health boost by topping them with spinach leaves and tomato, or spread your roll with smashed ripe avocado for additional healthy fats.

1. Cook the rice according to the package directions and set aside.

2. Heat 1 teaspoon of oil in a large nonstick skillet over medium heat. Add the carrots and onions and cook until the onions are translucent, about 4 minutes. Reduce the heat to low, cover, and continue cooking for 5 to 6 minutes, until the carrots are tender.

3. Add the beans and seasoning to the skillet and continue cooking for 2 to 3 more minutes.

4. Transfer the bean mixture to a food processor and wipe the skillet clean. Pulse the bean mixture 3 to 4 times or until the mixture is coarsely blended. Transfer the mixture to a medium bowl and fold in the brown rice until well combined.

5. Divide the mixture evenly and form it into 4 patties with your hands. Heat the remaining oil in the skillet. Cook the patties for 4 to 5 minutes per side, turning once.

6. Serve the burgers on the rolls with your choice of toppings.

**CONTINUED**

## Black Bean Burgers CONTINUED

**STORAGE TIP:** Store cooked burgers in the freezer for up to 3 months. You can reheat them directly from the freezer using a toaster oven or in a nonstick skillet.

. . . . . . . . . . . . . . . . . . . . . . . . . . . . . . . . . . . . . . . . . . . . . . . . . . . . .

**Per Serving (1 burger)**  Calories: 368; Total fat: 6g; Carbohydrates: 66g; Fiber: 8g; Protein: 13g; Calcium: 86mg; Sodium: 322mg; Potassium: 413mg; Vitamin D: 0mcg; Iron: 4mg; Zinc: 2mg

# Greek Flatbread with Spinach, Tomatoes & Feta

✔ **30 MINUTES OR LESS**
✔ **ONE-POT**
✔ **VEGETARIAN**

**SERVES 2**

**PREP TIME:** 10 MINUTES
**COOK TIME:** 9 MINUTES

2 cups fresh baby spinach, coarsely chopped

2 teaspoons olive oil

2 slices naan, or another flatbread

¼ cup sliced black olives

2 plum tomatoes, thinly sliced

1 teaspoon salt-free Italian seasoning blend

¼ cup crumbled feta

*Pizza.* The word conjures up decadent cheese-topped triangles and most likely lovely memories of time spent with friends. Pull these flatbreads together quickly and with no guilt when you're craving pizza. This version is lower in calories and sodium than a restaurant or frozen pie and includes heart-healthy monounsaturated fats, too. They can serve as an appetizer for a party or be paired with a green salad for dinner.

1. Preheat the oven to 400°F.

2. Heat 3 tablespoons of water in a small skillet over medium heat. Add the spinach, cover, and steam until wilted, about 2 minutes. Drain off any excess water and set aside.

3. Drizzle the oil evenly onto both flatbreads. Top each evenly with the spinach, olives, tomatoes, seasoning, and feta.

4. Bake the flatbreads directly on the oven rack for 5 to 7 minutes, or until lightly browned. Cut each into four pieces and serve hot.

**VARIATION TIP:** You can skip the cheese or use vegan cheese (and be sure to use a vegan flatbread, as most naan contains dairy or eggs) to make this dish vegan.

**STORAGE TIP:** Store leftovers in an airtight container in the refrigerator for up to 3 days.

. . . . . . . . . . . . . . . . . . . . . . . . . . . . . . . . . . . . . . . . . . . . . . .

**Per Serving** Calories: 411; Total fat: 15g; Carbohydrates: 53g; Fiber: 7g; Protein: 15g; Calcium: 191mg; Sodium: 621mg; Potassium: 522mg; Vitamin D: 0mcg; Iron: 3mg; Zinc: 2mg

# Mushroom Risotto with Peas

✔ 30 MINUTES OR LESS
✔ ONE-POT
✔ VEGETARIAN

**SERVES 2**

**PREP TIME:** 5 MINUTES
**COOK TIME:** 20 MINUTES

2 cups low-sodium vegetable or chicken broth

1 teaspoon olive oil

8 ounces baby portobello mushrooms, thinly sliced

½ cup frozen peas

1 teaspoon butter

1 cup arborio rice

1 tablespoon grated Parmesan cheese

Risotto is a culinary masterpiece created with arborio rice. The starchy quality of this ingredient creates the smooth and creamy texture of the dish. It's not difficult to produce, despite its intimidating reputation. Portobello mushrooms offer an array of B vitamins, and their umami factor helps boost flavors in low-salt cooking.

1. Pour the broth into a microwave-proof glass measuring cup. Microwave on high for 1½ minutes or until hot.

2. Heat the oil over medium heat in a large saucepan. Add the mushrooms and stir for 1 minute. Cover and cook until soft, about 3 more minutes. Stir in the peas and reduce the heat to low.

3. Move the mushroom mixture to the sides of the saucepan and add the butter to the middle, heating until melted. Add the rice to the saucepan and stir for 1 to 2 minutes to lightly toast. Add the hot broth, ½ cup at a time, and stir gently. As the broth is cooked into the rice, continue adding more broth, ½ cup at a time, stirring after each addition, until all broth is added. Once all of the liquid is absorbed (this should take 15 minutes), remove from the heat.

4. Serve immediately, topped with Parmesan cheese.

**SUBSTITUTION TIP:** If you don't have broth on hand, you can use white wine.

**STORAGE TIP:** Store the leftovers in an airtight container in the refrigerator for up to 3 days.

. . . . . . . . . . . . . . . . . . . . . . . . . . . . . . . . . . . . . . . . . . . . . . .

**Per Serving** Calories: 430; Total fat: 6g; Carbohydrates: 83g; Fiber: 5g; Protein: 10g; Calcium: 53mg; Sodium: 78mg; Potassium: 558mg; Vitamin D: 0mcg; Iron: 3mg; Zinc: 2mg

# Loaded Tofu Burrito with Black Beans

✔ **30 MINUTES OR LESS**
✔ **ONE-POT**
✔ **VEGETARIAN**

**SERVES 2**

**PREP TIME:** 5 MINUTES
**COOK TIME:** 20 MINUTES

4 ounces extra-firm tofu, pressed and cut into 2-inch cubes

2 teaspoons mesquite salt-free seasoning, divided

2 teaspoons canola oil

1 cup thinly sliced bell peppers

½ cup diced onions

⅔ cup black beans, drained and rinsed

2 (10-inch) whole-wheat tortillas

1 tablespoon sriracha

Nonfat Greek yogurt, for serving

Healthy eating does not usually include fat- and sodium-packed burritos, but this veggie-filled version will stand in nicely when your burrito craving hits. Quick and simple to make, it provides a satisfying, high-fiber meal. The secret to perfectly seared tofu is cooking it over medium heat in hot oil without turning until it's slightly crispy on the outside and lifts off easily.

1. Put the tofu and 1 teaspoon of seasoning in a medium zip-top plastic freezer bag and toss until the tofu is well coated.

2. Heat the oil in a medium skillet over medium-high heat. Add the tofu to the skillet. Don't stir; allow the tofu to brown before turning. When lightly browned all over, about 6 minutes, transfer the tofu from the skillet to a small bowl and set aside.

3. Add the peppers and onions to the skillet and sauté until tender, about 5 minutes. Reduce the heat to medium-low and add the beans and the remaining seasoning. Cook until the beans are heated through, about 5 minutes.

4. To assemble the burritos, lay each tortilla flat on a work surface. Place half of the tofu in the center of each tortilla, top with half of the pepper-bean mixture, and drizzle with the sriracha. Fold the bottom portion of each tortilla up and over the tofu mixture. Then fold each side into the middle, tuck in, and tightly roll it up toward the open end.

5. Serve with a dollop of yogurt.

**CONTINUED**

# Loaded Tofu Burrito with Black Beans CONTINUED

**PREP TIP:** For the crispiest results, press the moisture out of the tofu before cooking. Place the tofu on a paper towel-lined plate and place another paper towel and plate on top. Press gently until the liquid drains out.

. . . . . . . . . . . . . . . . . . . . . . . . . . . . . . . . . . . . . . . . . . . . . . . . . . . .

**Per Serving**  Calories: 327; Total fat: 12g; Carbohydrates: 41g; Fiber: 11g; Protein: 16g; Calcium: 230mg; Sodium: 282mg; Potassium: 568mg; Vitamin D: 0mcg; Iron: 3mg; Zinc: 2mg

# Fusilli Primavera

**SERVES 2**

**PREP TIME:** 10 MINUTES
**COOK TIME:** 20 MINUTES

### For the Pasta

2 teaspoons olive oil

1 garlic clove, pressed or minced

1 head broccoli, cut into small florets

1 large carrot, shaved into curls

1 large red bell pepper, thinly sliced

4 ounces fusilli pasta

### For the Sauce

2 teaspoons unsalted butter

1 tablespoon all-purpose flour

1 cup 1 percent milk

2 tablespoons light cream cheese

¼ cup grated Parmesan cheese, divided

### For the Toppings

½ cup part-skim ricotta

1 tablespoon chopped fresh parsley

Freshly ground black pepper

Primavera means "spring" in Italian and usually refers to a dish bursting with tender, colorful vegetables. Pasta is a perfect vehicle for showcasing vegetables. This dish is loaded with them and will help you meet your daily serving goals. You can really use any seasonal vegetable you like, but try to get an assortment of colors for visual impact.

## To Make the Pasta

1. Heat the oil in a medium skillet over medium heat. Add the garlic, stir for 1 minute, then add the broccoli florets and carrots and cook for 2 minutes. Reduce the heat to low and add the peppers, cover, and let steam for 2 minutes until the broccoli is bright green. Remove from the heat.

2. Fill a stockpot three-quarters full with water and bring it to a boil over high heat. Add the fusilli and cook al dente, 8 to 9 minutes.

## To Make the Sauce

3. Melt the butter in a large saucepan over medium heat. Whisk in the flour for 30 seconds until blended. Slowly pour in the milk, whisking constantly, until the sauce boils. Then reduce the heat to low, so the sauce simmers, and stir in the cream cheese until melted. Add 3 tablespoons of the Parmesan and stir until creamy and well blended.

4. Drain the pasta (do not rinse) and transfer it to the saucepan, stirring to coat the pasta with the sauce.

CONTINUED ▶

5. Transfer the pasta to two dishes. Top each with half of the vegetables, gently nestling them into the pasta. Garnish with the remaining cheese, ¼ cup ricotta each, and parsley.

6. Season to taste with pepper and serve.

PREP TIP: To shave carrot curls, simply use a potato peeler to peel carrots into short, thin strips. This allows them to cook more quickly and blend into the pasta dish.

STORAGE TIP: Store leftovers in an airtight container in the refrigerator for up to 3 days.

. . . . . . . . . . . . . . . . . . . . . . . . . . . . . . . . . . . . . . . . . . . . . . . . . .

Per Serving Calories: 664; Total fat: 23g; Carbohydrates: 87g; Fiber: 13g; Protein: 34g; Calcium: 629mg; Sodium: 528mg; Potassium: 1717mg; Vitamin D: 2mcg; Iron: 4mg; Zinc: 4mg

# Noodles with Mushrooms & Cabbage

✔ BUDGET-SAVER

✔ VEGETARIAN

**SERVES 2**

**PREP TIME:** 10 MINUTES
**COOK TIME:** 30 MINUTES

Pinch salt

1 tablespoon olive oil

4 ounces button
mushrooms, sliced

½ cup chopped onion

½ small head (about
3 cups) green or red
cabbage, thinly sliced

⅛ teaspoon
cayenne pepper

4 ounces wide whole-wheat
egg noodles

1 tablespoon
unsalted butter

Freshly ground
black pepper

Nonfat Greek
yogurt (optional)

Move over, kale! Cabbage is a budget-friendly, underrated cruciferous vegetable that's loaded with Vitamin C and other antioxidants. It can help you keep your digestive system in check and lower your cholesterol, too. This recipe is a comfort dish with Hungarian roots; by adding mushrooms and reducing the butter, this meal becomes DASH-approved.

1. Fill a large saucepan three-quarters full with water, add the salt, and bring it to a boil over high heat.

2. While the water is coming to a boil, heat the oil in a medium skillet over medium heat. Add the mushrooms and onion and sauté for 4 minutes. Add the cabbage and cayenne pepper, cover, and cook for 10 to 15 minutes or until cabbage is tender.

3. Add the noodles to the boiling water and cook until al dente, about 8 minutes, or according to package directions.

4. Drain the noodles and transfer them to a serving dish. Top the noodles with the butter and toss to coat. Top the noodles with the cabbage and mushrooms, tossing together gently. Season with pepper.

5. Serve topped with a dollop of yogurt (if using).

**SUBSTITUTION TIP:** You can also use pappardelle noodles in place of egg noodles.

. . . . . . . . . . . . . . . . . . . . . . . . . . . . . . . . . . . . . . . . . . . . . . . . . . . .

**Per Serving** Calories: 381; Total fat: 14g; Carbohydrates: 59g; Fiber: 10g; Protein: 13g; Calcium: 107mg; Sodium: 120mg; Potassium: 668mg; Vitamin D: 0mcg; Iron: 3mg; Zinc: 2mg

# Simple Spinach Frittata

✔ **30 MINUTES OR LESS**

✔ **VEGETARIAN**

**SERVES 2**

**PREP TIME:** 5 MINUTES
**COOK TIME:** 20 MINUTES

4 large eggs

¼ cup 1 percent milk

¼ cup part-skim ricotta

¼ teaspoon Herbs de Provence

Pinch freshly ground black pepper

Pinch salt

1 teaspoon olive oil

1 shallot, finely chopped

2 cups fresh baby spinach

It's always a good idea to have a dozen eggs in the refrigerator for a quick meal, such as this frittata. Eggs are versatile and provide 13 important nutrients, including choline, lutein, and Vitamin D. Plus, an egg has only 70 calories. Although eggs are delicious, spinach is the real star of this dish. The deep green flecks throughout are gorgeous, and the earthy taste is perfect with the mild, slightly tart ricotta and French-themed herbs.

1. Preheat the oven to 400°F.

2. In a small bowl, stir together the eggs, milk, ricotta, herbs, pepper, and salt until well mixed. Set aside.

3. Heat the oil in a medium oven-safe skillet over medium heat. Add the shallot and cook for 1 to 2 minutes. Add the spinach and stir until wilted, about 4 minutes.

4. Pour the egg mixture into the skillet and stir gently. Reduce the heat to low and allow the eggs to set.

5. To finish cooking, place the skillet in the oven for 5 to 10 minutes or until the eggs are completely set and lightly browned.

6. Remove the frittata from the oven and loosen the bottom with a spatula. Carefully invert the frittata onto a plate and serve.

**VARIATION TIP:** Swap in chopped asparagus or peppers in place of the spinach for another great option.

**STORAGE TIP:** Store leftovers in an airtight container in the refrigerator for up to 3 days.

· · · · · · · · · · · · · · · · · · · · · · · · · · · · · · · · · · · · · · · · · · · · · · · · · · · · · · · · · · · · · · · · · · · · · · · · · · · · · · · · · · · ·

**Per Serving** Calories: 229; Total fat: 15g; Carbohydrates: 6g; Fiber: 1g; Protein: 18g; Calcium: 210mg; Sodium: 288mg; Potassium: 407mg; Vitamin D: 2mcg; Iron: 3mg; Zinc: 2mg

# Sugar Snap Noodles with Gingered Pesto

**SERVES 2**

**PREP TIME:** 20 MINUTES
**COOK TIME:** 15 MINUTES

**For the Ginger Pesto**

1½ cups fresh baby spinach

¼ cup packed basil leaves

2 tablespoons
  chopped walnuts

2 tablespoons grated
  Parmesan cheese

1 teaspoon peeled and
  grated fresh ginger

2 garlic cloves, minced

Juice of ½ lemon

2 tablespoons olive oil

**For the Noodles**

4 ounces spaghetti

1 cup sugar snap peas

1 cup shredded carrots

1 cup shelled
  frozen edamame

Edamame is the Japanese name for immature (green) soybeans. This humble ingredient provides 8 grams of protein per half cup, adding incredible nutrition oomph to this veggie pasta dish. The pesto is pumped up with spinach and has a kick from the fresh ginger. I use walnuts in place of pine nuts because they are less expensive and easier to find, but feel free to substitute any nuts you might have on hand. If you're short on time, you can use a jarred pesto, but it will be higher in sodium, so be sure to check the label.

## To Make the Ginger Pesto

1. Put the spinach, basil, walnuts, Parmesan cheese, ginger, garlic, and lemon juice in a food processor. Pulse until well chopped.

2. Gradually add the olive oil by the spoonful, pulsing after each addition, until the mixture becomes a smooth paste. Set aside.

## To Make the Noodles

3. Fill a large stockpot three-quarters full with water and bring it to a boil over high heat.

4. Add the pasta and set a timer to cook for 8 minutes.

5. After the pasta has been cooking for 6 minutes, add the snap peas, carrots, and edamame to the pot.

6. Drain the pasta and vegetables and transfer them to a serving bowl. Add the pesto, toss to coat, and serve.

CONTINUED ▶

Sugar Snap Noodles with Gingered Pesto CONTINUED

**SUBSTITUTION TIP:** You can substitute ¼ teaspoon ground ginger in place of the 1 teaspoon fresh ginger.

**STORAGE TIP:** Store leftovers in an airtight container in the refrigerator for up to 3 days.

. . . . . . . . . . . . . . . . . . . . . . . . . . . . . . . . . . . . . . . . . . . . . .

**Per Serving**  Calories: 560; Total fat: 25g; Carbohydrates: 65g; Fiber: 11g; Protein: 22g; Calcium: 199mg; Sodium: 158mg; Potassium: 983mg; Vitamin D: 0mcg; Iron: 6mg; Zinc: 3mg

# Sweet Potato Rice with Spicy Peanut Sauce

✔ ONE-POT

✔ VEGAN

**SERVES 2**

**PREP TIME:** 20 MINUTES
**COOK TIME:** 25 MINUTES

½ cup basmati rice

2 teaspoons olive oil, divided

1 (8-ounce) can chickpeas, drained and rinsed

2 medium sweet potatoes, peeled and cut into small cubes

¼ teaspoon ground cumin

1 cup water

⅛ teaspoon salt

2 tablespoons chopped cilantro

3 tablespoons peanut butter

1 tablespoon sriracha

2 teaspoons reduced-sodium soy sauce

½ teaspoon garlic powder

¼ teaspoon ground ginger

This simple rice dish is packed with brightly hued sweet potatoes and fiber-rich beans. Sweet potatoes are high in vitamin A and potassium. The beans provide some extra protein, some iron, and additional potassium. When you top it with the spicy peanut sauce, this one-bowl meal has a delightfully complex flavor reminiscent of Pad Thai.

1. Rinse the rice in a mesh strainer under cold water and set it aside.

2. Heat 1 teaspoon of oil in a large nonstick skillet over medium-high heat. Add the chickpeas and heat for 3 minutes. Stir and cook until lightly browned. Transfer the chickpeas to a small bowl. Add the remaining 1 teaspoon of oil to the skillet, then add the potatoes and cumin, distributing them evenly. Cook the potatoes until they become lightly browned before turning them.

3. While the potatoes are cooking, boil the water with the salt in a large saucepan over medium-high heat. Add the rice to the boiling water, reduce the heat to low, cover, and simmer for 20 minutes or until the water is absorbed.

4. When the potatoes have fully cooked, about 10 minutes in total, remove the skillet from the heat. Transfer the potatoes and chickpeas to the rice, folding all together gently. Add the chopped cilantro.

**CONTINUED** ▶

5. In a small bowl, whisk together the peanut butter, sriracha, soy sauce, garlic powder, and ginger until well blended.

6. Divide the rice mixture between two serving bowls. Drizzle with the sauce and serve.

**SUBSTITUTION TIP:** You can substitute frozen butternut squash for the sweet potatoes.

**INGREDIENT TIP:** Rinsing the rice helps remove starch so it doesn't become too sticky for this dish.

. . . . . . . . . . . . . . . . . . . . . . . . . . . . . . . . . . . . . . . . . . . . .

**Per Serving** Calories: 667; Total fat: 22g; Carbohydrates: 100g; Fiber: 14g; Protein: 20g; Calcium: 109mg; Sodium: 563mg; Potassium: 963mg; Vitamin D: 0mcg; Iron: 7mg; Zinc: 3mg

# Vegetable Red Curry

**SERVES 2**

**PREP TIME:** 15 MINUTES
**COOK TIME:** 25 MINUTES

2 teaspoons olive oil

1 cup sliced carrots

½ cup chopped onion

1 garlic clove, pressed
  or minced

2 bell peppers, seeded and
  thinly sliced

1 cup chopped cauliflower

⅔ cup light coconut milk

½ cup low-sodium
  vegetable broth

1 tablespoon tomato paste

1 teaspoon curry powder

½ teaspoon ground cumin

½ teaspoon
  ground coriander

¼ teaspoon turmeric

2 cups fresh baby spinach

1 cup quick-cooking
  brown rice

Curry is an easy weeknight meal to make, and the abundant spices allow you to skip the salt without losing an iota of flavor. This dish uses regular vegetable broth, so if you do use a reduced-sodium broth, you can add a pinch of salt. This main dish is super-packed with veggies, so it will satisfy four servings of DASH vegetables for the day.

1. Heat the oil in a large nonstick skillet over medium heat. Add the carrots, onion, and garlic and cook for 2 to 3 minutes.

2. Reduce the heat to medium-low, add the peppers and cauliflower to the skillet, cover, and cook for about 5 minutes until the vegetables are tender.

3. Add the coconut milk, broth, tomato paste, curry powder, cumin, coriander, and turmeric, stirring to combine. Simmer, covered (vent the lid slightly), for 10 to 15 minutes until the curry is slightly reduced and thickened. Uncover, add the spinach, and stir for 2 minutes until it is wilted and mixed into the vegetables. Remove from the heat.

4. While the vegetables are cooking, cook the rice according to the package instructions.

5. Serve the curry over the rice.

**VARIATION TIP:** For an extra protein boost, in step 2, you can add an 8-ounce can of chickpeas, drained and rinsed.

**STORAGE TIP:** Store leftovers in an airtight container in the refrigerator for up to 3 days.

. . . . . . . . . . . . . . . . . . . . . . . . . . . . . . . . . . . . . . . . . . . . . .

**Per Serving** Calories: 584; Total fat: 16g; Carbohydrates: 101g; Fiber: 10g; Protein: 13g; Calcium: 146mg; Sodium: 102mg; Potassium: 1430mg; Vitamin D: 0mcg; Iron: 6mg; Zinc: 3mg

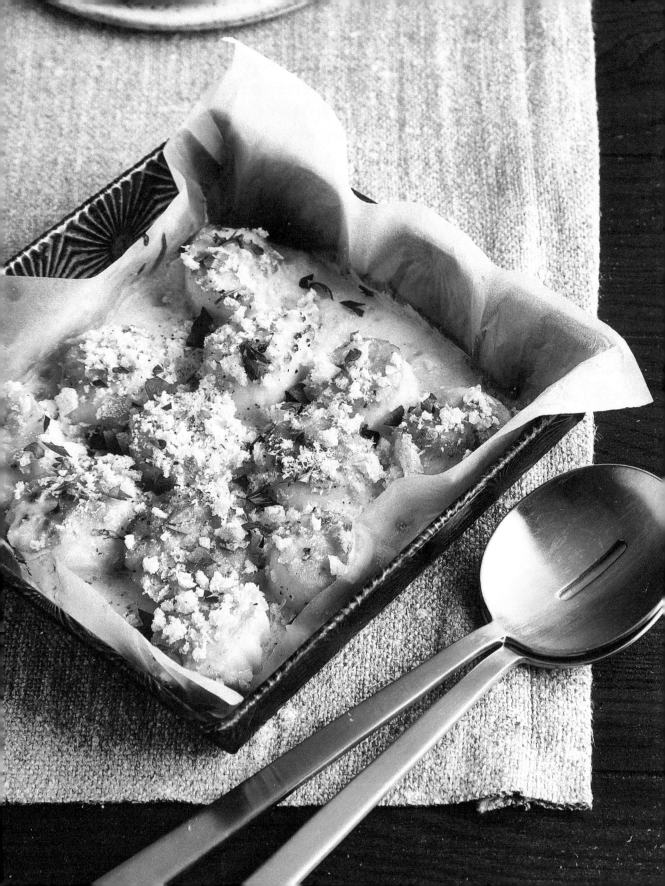

# 6

# FISH AND SEAFOOD

# Shrimp & Broccoli with Angel Hair

✔ 30 MINUTES OR LESS
✔ ONE-POT

**SERVES 2**

**PREP TIME:** 10 MINUTES
**COOK TIME:** 15 MINUTES

Pinch salt

4 teaspoons olive oil, divided

1 garlic clove, pressed or minced

1 broccoli head, cut into florets

12 frozen, cooked large shrimp, peeled, deveined, and tails removed

4 ounces angel hair pasta

2 tablespoons Parmesan cheese

Freshly ground black pepper (optional)

This pasta dish is made with common ingredients found in most kitchens. You can use frozen broccoli in place of fresh and can add other vegetables, too. The dish comes together quickly thanks to frozen cooked shrimp and quick-cooking angel hair pasta, making it a go-to dish for busy evenings. While shrimp is higher in cholesterol than chicken or beef, it's very low in saturated fat and fits into a DASH meal plan.

1. Fill a large stockpot three-quarters full with water, add the salt, and bring it to a boil over high heat.

2. Heat 1 teaspoon of oil in a medium skillet over medium-high heat. Add the garlic and cook for 1 minute. Add the broccoli and sauté for 3 to 4 minutes. Cover and let the vegetables steam for an additional 2 minutes. The broccoli should be bright green and fork-tender. Set aside off the heat.

3. Add the angel hair to the boiling water and cook for 2 to 4 minutes, according to the directions on the package. Drain and immediately add to the skillet. Add the remaining 1 tablespoon of olive oil and stir. Return to low heat to heat through, about 3 minutes.

4. Divide the pasta between two dishes and garnish with the Parmesan cheese and pepper to taste (if using).

**INGREDIENT TIP:** Angel hair pasta cooks very quickly, so be careful not to overcook it!

. . . . . . . . . . . . . . . . . . . . . . . . . . . . . . . . . . . . . . . . . . . . .

**Per Serving** Calories: 456; Total fat: 12g; Carbohydrates: 64g; Fiber: 10g; Protein: 25g; Calcium: 230mg; Sodium: 583mg; Potassium: 1158mg; Vitamin D: 0mcg; Iron: 4mg; Zinc: 3mg

# Maple-Glazed Salmon

✓ ONE-POT

**SERVES 2**

**PREP TIME:** 15 MINUTES
**COOK TIME:** 20 MINUTES

2 (5- to 6-ounce) salmon
fillets, skin-on

½ teaspoon salt-free
mesquite seasoning

1 tablespoon pure
maple syrup

The beauty of fish is that it cooks quickly and tastes like you spent hours creating it. This maple-glazed salmon provides heart-healthy omega-3 fatty acids and protein. Whenever possible, use pure maple syrup even though it can be pricey, because the flavor is exceptional and a little goes a long way. Serve this fish with a side of Garlicky Roasted Broccoli (page 163) or Sautéed Zucchini with Onions (page 164).

1. Preheat the oven to 425°F. Line a baking sheet with parchment paper or a silicone mat.

2. Place the salmon onto the baking sheet (skin side down) and rub the seasoning evenly over each fillet. Drizzle the syrup onto the fillets, rubbing to coat the top.

3. Put the baking sheet in the oven and bake for 15 to 20 minutes.

4. Serve.

**COOKING TIP:** An oven-style air fryer gives the salmon a slightly crisp outer layer while keeping it moist inside. Line the air-fryer pan with foil, place the salmon on it as in step 2, put it in the oven, and air fry for 5 to 8 minutes, checking to be sure the salmon doesn't overcook.

. . . . . . . . . . . . . . . . . . . . . . . . . . . . . . . . . . . . . . . . . . . . . .

**Per Serving** Calories: 223; Total fat: 9g; Carbohydrates: 7g; Fiber: 0g; Protein: 28g; Calcium: 27mg; Sodium: 64mg; Potassium: 716mg; Vitamin D: 9mcg; Iron: 1mg; Zinc: 1mg

# Tilapia Tacos with Chipotle Cream

✔ 30 MINUTES OR LESS
✔ ONE-POT

**SERVES 2**

**PREP TIME:** 5 MINUTES
**COOK TIME:** 10 MINUTES

**For the Tacos**

1 teaspoon olive oil

10 to 12 ounces tilapia

1 teaspoon chili powder

½ teaspoon ground cumin

⅛ teaspoon salt

4 (6-inch) flour tortillas

**For the Sauce**

½ teaspoon
  smoked paprika

¼ teaspoon cayenne
  pepper, or to taste

½ cup nonfat Greek yogurt

1 chipotle pepper in adobo
  sauce, chopped

Taco Tuesday is even better with these lower sodium fish tacos. Creating your own taco seasoning adds flavor without the extra unhealthy ingredients. The tilapia cooks up in a skillet so quickly that you can have lunch or dinner on the table in fewer than 20 minutes. Serve these with cabbage slaw, a green salad, or another vegetable to round out the meal.

### To Make the Tacos

1. Heat the oil in a medium skillet on medium-high heat. Add the tilapia to the hot skillet and sprinkle it with the chili powder, cumin, and salt. Cook for 3 to 4 minutes per side. Remove the fish from the heat and gently flake it into bite-size pieces.

2. Wrap the tortillas in a paper towel and heat them for 1 minute in the microwave on high.

### To Make the Sauce

3. In a small bowl, mix together the paprika and cayenne pepper. Add the yogurt and chopped chipotle pepper to the spices, blending well.

4. Divide the fish between the tortillas, top with a spoon of the chipotle cream, and serve.

**VARIATION TIP:** To make a thicker taco sauce for the fish, mix the chili powder, cumin, and salt with ¼ teaspoon of cornstarch. Add this mixture and ¼ cup water to the skillet in step 1.

. . . . . . . . . . . . . . . . . . . . . . . . . . . . . . . . . . . . . . . . .

**Per Serving** Calories: 383; Total fat: 9g; Carbohydrates: 36g; Fiber: 3g; Protein: 40g; Calcium: 168mg; Sodium: 716mg; Potassium: 727mg; Vitamin D: 2mcg; Iron: 4mg; Zinc: 1mg

# Baked Haddock with Peppers & Eggplant

✔ 30 MINUTES OR LESS

**SERVES 2 TO 3**

**PREP TIME:** 15 MINUTES
**COOK TIME:** 20 MINUTES

Nonstick cooking spray

2 (5- to 6-ounce)
 haddock fillets

½ teaspoon salt-free
 Italian seasoning

1 teaspoon olive oil

2 garlic cloves, pressed
 or minced

½ cup diced onion

5 to 6 mini bell
 peppers, chopped

1 small eggplant, peeled
 and diced

6 large green olives, pitted
 and sliced

2 tablespoons
 tomato paste

2 tablespoons
 balsamic vinegar

1 tablespoon
 granulated sugar

This low-calorie dish is inspired by caponata, a sweet-and-sour Italian dish composed of tomato, pepper, and eggplant. In addition to the fish, you'll get two servings of vegetables in this meal, as well as good amounts of healthy fats, vitamin C, potassium, and fiber.

1. Preheat the oven to 375°F. Spray a 9-by-11-inch baking dish with cooking spray. Place the fish in the prepared baking dish, sprinkle it with the seasoning, and bake for 15 or 20 minutes, until opaque.

2. Meanwhile, in a large saucepan, heat the oil over medium heat. Add the garlic and cook for 1 minute. Add the onion and cook for 2 to 3 minutes.

3. Add the peppers and eggplant. Reduce the heat to low, cover, and allow the vegetables to steam until tender, about 6 minutes. Add a few spoons of water if needed.

4. Add the olives, tomato paste, vinegar, and sugar to the eggplant mixture and stir to combine. If needed, add a few more spoonfuls of water. Cover and simmer for 10 minutes, stirring occasionally.

5. To serve, top each serving of fish with ¾ cup of the caponata.

**STORAGE TIP:** Store leftover caponata in the refrigerator for up to a week. It can be served as a side dish, on top of pasta, or spread on toasted bread as a snack.

. . . . . . . . . . . . . . . . . . . . . . . . . . . . . . . . . . . . . . . . . .

**Per Serving** Calories: 357; Total fat: 6g; Carbohydrates: 51g; Fiber: 13g; Protein: 30g; Calcium: 107mg; Sodium: 425mg; Potassium: 1876mg; Vitamin D: 0mcg; Iron: 3mg; Zinc: 2mg

# Creamy Italian-Style Sea Scallops

✔ MAKE-AHEAD

**SERVES 4**

**PREP TIME:** 45 MINUTES
**COOK TIME:** 30 MINUTES

### For the Scallops

½ teaspoon
  butter, softened

¾ cup dry white wine

1 medium onion, chopped

1 bay leaf

2 pounds sea scallops,
  thawed if frozen

### For the Sauce

2 tablespoons
  unsalted butter

1½ tablespoons
  all-purpose flour

¾ cup 1 percent milk

Dash salt

Freshly ground
  black pepper

¼ cup shredded
  fontina cheese

1 tablespoon bread crumbs

¼ cup grated
  Parmesan cheese

This is an elegant, company-worthy meal of succulent, tender scallops baked in a cheesy sauce and topped with golden bread crumbs. The classic milk-based white sauce is not only versatile but is a great way to get your DASH servings of dairy in. This version is also much lower in fat than traditional cream sauces, and the wine reduction adds incredibly rich flavor.

## To Make the Scallops

*1.* Grease an 8-by-8-inch baking dish with the butter.

*2.* Stir together the wine, onion, and bay leaf in a small saucepan. Bring to a boil over high heat, reduce the heat to low, and simmer until the liquid is reduced by half, about 4 to 5 minutes.

*3.* Strain the liquid into a measuring cup. Carefully wipe the saucepan clean with a paper towel. Save the onions for another use, discard the bay leaf, and set the wine stock aside.

*4.* Sauté the scallops in a large nonstick skillet over medium heat, for 5 to 7 minutes, or until their liquid is released. Drain. Place the scallops in the baking dish and set aside.

*5.* Preheat the oven to 400°F.

## To Make the Sauce

*6.* Melt the butter in the small saucepan over medium-low heat, add the flour, and whisk for 1 minute.

*7.* Reduce the heat to low, and immediately add the milk and wine stock. Whisk constantly until smooth and thick. Season with the salt and pepper to taste.

8. Add the shredded fontina cheese and stir until the cheese is melted and the sauce is creamy, about 2 minutes. Remove the sauce from the heat.

9. Pour the sauce over the scallops. Sprinkle them with the bread crumbs and Parmesan cheese.

10. Bake for 15 minutes, until bubbly and lightly browned, and serve.

**SUBSTITUTION TIP:** If you don't like scallops, substitute chicken breast.

**STORAGE TIP:** Store leftovers in a sealed container in the refrigerator for up to 3 days.

. . . . . . . . . . . . . . . . . . . . . . . . . . . . . . . . . . . . . . . . . . . . . . . . . .

**Per Serving** Calories: 342; Total fat: 12g; Carbohydrates: 16g; Fiber: 1g; Protein: 33g; Calcium: 174mg; Sodium: 423mg; Potassium: 625mg; Vitamin D: 1mcg; Iron: 1mg; Zinc: 3mg

# Tex-Mex Cod with Roasted Peppers & Corn

✔ ONE-POT

**SERVES 2**

**PREP TIME:** 10 MINUTES
**COOK TIME:** 30 MINUTES

6 mini bell peppers, assorted colors, quartered

1 cup frozen corn

2 teaspoons olive oil, divided

1 tablespoon salt-free Tex-Mex or mesquite seasoning, divided

Nonstick cooking spray

2 (6- to 8-ounce) haddock fillets

1 lime, quartered

¼ cup plain Greek yogurt, seasoned with ¼ teaspoon salt-free Tex-Mex seasoning (optional)

This is a speedy sheet-pan meal. The fish roasts alongside the peppers and corn, giving the dish its rich, smoky flavor. When you layer extra vegetables onto the baking sheet, you build more flavor and texture, allowing you to use less salt. This meal comes together quickly, and its kitchen clean-up is minimal.

1. Preheat the oven to 425°F. Line a baking sheet with parchment paper or a silicone mat.

2. Spread the peppers and corn evenly over two-thirds of the baking sheet. Drizzle 1 teaspoon of oil over the vegetables, then sprinkle them with 2 teaspoons of the seasoning. Put the vegetables in the oven for 10 minutes to begin roasting. Remove baking sheet from the oven.

3. While the vegetables roast, spray a sheet of aluminum foil with cooking spray and place the fish on it. Drizzle the fish with the remaining oil and season it with the remaining 1 teaspoon of seasoning. Squeeze one lime wedge onto each fillet. Fold up the edges of the foil so the juices don't escape and transfer the fish to the baking sheet with the vegetables.

4. Return the baking sheet to the oven and bake for an additional 15 to 20 minutes until the fish is opaque white and flaky and the vegetables are tender and lightly charred.

**5.** Place a fish fillet on each plate, and top each with half of the roasted vegetables. Serve with a dollop of seasoned yogurt (if using).

INGREDIENT TIP: Tex-Mex seasoning generally contains chili powder, cumin, and pepper. If you can't find a salt-free blend, make your own using 1 tablespoon chili powder, 1 teaspoon ground cumin, 1 teaspoon paprika, and 1 teaspoon oregano.

. . . . . . . . . . . . . . . . . . . . . . . . . . . . . . . . . . . . . . . . . . . . . . . . . . . . .

**Per Serving** Calories: 340; Total fat: 7g; Carbohydrates: 38g; Fiber: 5g; Protein: 36g; Calcium: 84mg; Sodium: 382mg; Potassium: 1316mg; Vitamin D: 1mcg; Iron: 2mg; Zinc: 2mg

# Marinated Lime Grilled Shrimp

✔ ONE-POT

**SERVES 2**

**PREP TIME:** 10 MINUTES,
PLUS AT LEAST 30 MINUTES
TO MARINATE
**COOK TIME:** 10 MINUTES

1 lime, quartered, divided

¼ cup chopped fresh
  cilantro, divided

1 tablespoon rice
  wine vinegar

1 teaspoon avocado oil

¼ teaspoon chili powder

¼ teaspoon garlic powder

6 large shrimp, peeled
  and deveined

This light and fresh dish is spectacular all year round, but
it is especially delicious during warmer months when the
grill is available. This spicy lime and chili marinated shrimp
dish also makes a great appetizer or can be whipped up as
a special snack for the big game or a festive get-together.
Marinating the shrimp infuses a lot of the flavor, so be
sure to allow at least 30 minutes of marinating time. Serve
with Sweet Potato Steak Fries (page 172) or on top of a
green salad.

1. In a small bowl, mix together the juice from three lime
   quarters, 3 tablespoons cilantro, and the vinegar, oil,
   chili powder, and garlic powder.

2. Place the shrimp in the bowl with the marinade, toss to
   coat, and refrigerate it for 30 minutes or up to 4 hours.

3. Preheat a grill to medium-high. Place the shrimp on a
   grill pan and cook for 3 to 5 minutes, until white, turning once. Discard the marinade.

4. If you do not have a grill, pan-sear the shrimp in a
   nonstick skillet for 3 to 4 minutes, turning once.

5. Serve the shrimp with a squeeze of juice from the last
   lime quarter and the remaining cilantro.

**SUBSTITUTION TIP:** You can substitute apple cider vinegar for the rice wine vinegar. You can also use ½ teaspoon
of a salt-free seasoning blend to replace the chili and
garlic powders.

. . . . . . . . . . . . . . . . . . . . . . . . . . . . . . . . . . . . . . . . . . . . . . . . . . .

**Per Serving** Calories: 44; Total fat: 2g; Carbohydrates: 3g;
Fiber: 0g; Protein: 3g; Calcium: 18mg; Sodium: 131mg;
Potassium: 74mg; Vitamin D: 0mcg; Iron: 0 mg; Zinc: 0mg

# Saucy Penne with Shrimp, Peas & Walnuts

✔ **30 MINUTES OR LESS**

**SERVES 2**

**PREP TIME:** 5 MINUTES
**COOK TIME:** 20 MINUTES

1 teaspoon olive oil

12 large cooked frozen shrimp (peeled and deveined), thawed

1 cup frozen peas

½ cup chopped walnuts

½ teaspoon salt-free Italian seasoning blend

2 teaspoons unsalted butter

1 tablespoon all-purpose flour

1 cup 1 percent milk

2 tablespoons light cream cheese

¼ cup grated Parmesan cheese, divided

4 ounces penne pasta

Freshly ground black pepper

Pasta is a popular meal in most households, and many people make it once a week because it is so quick and easy. This unusual penne creation features tender shrimp, bright peas, and protein-packed walnuts in a creamy cheese sauce. The combination of ingredients is delicious and provides a partial serving of dairy and some extra healthy fat from the walnuts. Win-win!

1. Fill a large stockpot three-quarters full with water and bring it to a boil on high heat.

2. In a medium saucepan, heat the oil over medium-high heat and sauté the shrimp, peas, walnuts, and seasoning for 3 to 4 minutes. (Make sure any liquid from the shrimp is evaporated.) Transfer the mixture to a small bowl.

3. Wipe out the saucepan with a paper towel and melt the butter in it over medium heat. Whisk in the flour for 1 minute. Slowly pour in the milk and bring it to a boil, whisking occasionally. Reduce the heat to low, simmer, and stir in the cream cheese until it melts, about 3 minutes. Add 3 tablespoons of the Parmesan cheese and continue stirring until the sauce is creamy and well-blended, about 2 minutes. Add more milk if the sauce gets too thick. Remove it from the heat.

4. When the water is boiling, add the penne and boil for 8 to 9 minutes (or follow the package directions for al dente).

**CONTINUED** ▶

**5.** Drain the pasta and add it to the sauce. Stir to combine. Transfer the pasta to a serving dish and top it with the shrimp mixture. Garnish the pasta with the remaining Parmesan cheese, season it with pepper, and serve.

**SUBSTITUTION TIP:** You can use fresh shrimp and cook them for 4 to 5 minutes in step 2.

**STORAGE TIP:** Store any leftovers in the refrigerator for up to 3 days.

. . . . . . . . . . . . . . . . . . . . . . . . . . . . . . . . . . . . . . . . . . . . . . . . . . .

**Per Serving** Calories: 673; Total fat: 34g; Carbohydrates: 64g; Fiber: 6g; Protein: 31g; Calcium: 390mg; Sodium: 653mg; Potassium: 698mg; Vitamin D: 1mcg; Iron: 3mg; Zinc: 4mg

# Angel Hair with Smoked Salmon & Asparagus

✔ **30 MINUTES OR LESS**

**SERVES 2**

**PREP TIME:** 15 MINUTES
**COOK TIME:** 15 MINUTES

20 asparagus spears, trimmed and cut into 2-inch pieces

2 tablespoons olive oil, divided

4 ounces angel hair pasta

2 ounces smoked salmon, cut into bite-size pieces

1 teaspoon capers

2 tablespoons grated Parmesan cheese

Freshly ground black pepper

Delicate angel hair pasta pairs beautifully with thinly sliced smoked salmon and slender asparagus to create this light and elegant dish. Smoked salmon is higher in sodium than fresh fish, but it's delicious and helps make preparing this meal even faster. Low in saturated fat and high in protein, smoked salmon provides vitamins B and D, magnesium, and omega-3 fatty acids. It's widely available, and you can purchase it in small packages, making it ideal for cooking for two.

1. Fill a large stockpot three-quarters full with water and bring it to a boil over high heat.

2. Add 2 tablespoons of water to a large nonstick skillet over medium heat. When the water is simmering, add the asparagus, cover, and steam for 6 minutes. Remove the lid, drain off any remaining water, add 1½ teaspoons oil, and sauté for 1 to 2 more minutes.

3. Add the angel hair pasta to the boiling water and cook for 3 minutes (or according to the package directions). Drain the pasta, transfer it to a serving bowl, and add the asparagus, smoked salmon, the remaining 1½ tablespoons oil, and the capers and toss gently.

4. Serve topped with the Parmesan cheese and seasoned to taste with pepper.

**STORAGE TIP:** Store leftovers in an airtight container in the refrigerator for up to 3 days.

. . . . . . . . . . . . . . . . . . . . . . . . . . . . . . . . . . . . . . . . . . . . .

**Per Serving** Calories: 416; Total fat: 17g; Carbohydrates: 49g; Fiber: 5g; Protein: 18g; Calcium: 97mg; Sodium: 320mg; Potassium: 509mg; Vitamin D: 5mcg; Iron: 6mg; Zinc: 2mg

# Bass with Citrus Butter

✔ **30 MINUTES OR LESS**

✔ **ONE-POT**

**SERVES 2**

**PREP TIME:** 15 MINUTES
**COOK TIME:** 15 MINUTES

2 (5- to 7-ounce) bass
fillets, skin-on

1 teaspoon salt-free
seafood seasoning

⅛ teaspoon salt

1 lime, halved

1 tablespoon avocado
oil, divided

1 teaspoon butter

¼ teaspoon cumin

¼ cup slivered,
blanched almonds

Bass is a delicious, light fish and lends itself to citrusy
flavors. Unlike meatier fish, bass flakes into moist chunks
that you can coat with this luscious, buttery sauce. Any
whitefish would work beautifully with this light and fresh
sauce. Don't worry about overindulging; by blending the
butter with avocado oil, you reduce the total saturated fat in
the meal but still get the delicious flavor profile of butter.

1. Season the fish with the seasoning blend and salt.

2. In a microwave-safe glass measuring cup, stir together
   the juice of half a lime, 2 teaspoons oil, butter, and
   cumin until blended. Set aside.

3. Heat a large nonstick skillet over medium heat. Add the
   almonds and toast for 2 to 3 minutes, being careful they
   don't over-brown. Transfer the almonds to a small bowl
   and set aside.

4. Heat the remaining oil in the skillet over medium-
   high heat. Add the bass fillets, skin side up. Sear for
   3 minutes without disturbing the fillets, then turn them
   and finish cooking for another 3 to 4 minutes.

5. While the fish is searing, heat the citrus butter sauce for
   20 seconds in the microwave.

6. Transfer the fish to a serving dish, pour the citrus butter
   over it, and top it with the toasted almonds. Garnish
   with the remaining lime half cut into wedges and serve.

**PREP TIP:** You can toast the almonds in a skillet in a 350°F
oven for 5 minutes.

. . . . . . . . . . . . . . . . . . . . . . . . . . . . . . . . . . . . . . . . . . . . . . . . . . . . . . . .

**Per Serving** Calories: 325; Total fat: 21g; Carbohydrates: 5g;
Fiber: 2g; Protein: 30g; Calcium: 156mg; Sodium: 270mg;
Potassium: 634mg; Vitamin D: 13mcg; Iron: 3mg; Zinc: 1mg

# Seared Mahi-Mahi with Lemon & Parsley

✔ ONE-POT

**SERVES 2**

**PREP TIME:** 20 MINUTES, PLUS AT LEAST 15 MINUTES TO MARINATE
**COOK TIME:** 15 MINUTES

2 teaspoons avocado oil

Juice of ½ lemon

½ teaspoon oregano

½ teaspoon garlic powder

¼ teaspoon Worcestershire sauce

2 (5- to 7-ounce) mahi-mahi steaks

1 tablespoon chopped parsley

½ lemon, cut into two wedges

Mahi-mahi is also known as dorado or dolphinfish, but it's not a dolphin! It may get that name due to its large dorsal fin. This mild, flaky fish is common in the Gulf of Mexico and has a mild, sweet flavor profile. Like all fish, this protein cooks up in minutes. You can prep the marinade early in the day to save time at mealtime.

1. Preheat the oven to 400°F. (If you'll be marinating the fish for longer than 15 minutes, preheat the oven just before baking.) Line a baking sheet with parchment paper or a silicone mat.

2. In a medium bowl, stir together the oil, lemon juice, oregano, garlic powder, and Worcestershire sauce. Put the fish in a medium zip-top plastic bag and add the marinade. Press out any excess air, seal the bag, and marinate the fish in the refrigerator for 15 minutes or up to 2 hours.

3. Remove the fish from the marinade, place it on the prepared baking sheet, and roast it for 15 minutes (discard the marinade).

4. To serve, garnish each mahi-mahi steak with parsley and a lemon wedge.

**PREP TIP:** Make this a sheet-pan meal. Place small potatoes and sliced zucchini (½-inch slices) on one side of a baking sheet and drizzle them with olive oil. Bake in a 400°F oven for 25 minutes, and then add the fish, roasting for 15 more minutes.

..................................................

**Per Serving** Calories: 282; Total fat: 18g; Carbohydrates: 3g; Fiber: g; Protein: 26g; Calcium: 41mg; Sodium: 101mg; Potassium: 594mg; Vitamin D: 16mcg; Iron: 1mg; Zinc: 1mg

# Pan-Fried Crusted Salmon with Mustard Panko

✓ **30 MINUTES OR LESS**

✓ **ONE-POT**

**SERVES 2**

**PREP TIME:** 5 MINUTES

**COOK TIME:** 10 MINUTES

1 tablespoon Dijon mustard

1 tablespoon light
  sour cream

2 skinless salmon fillets
  (5 to 6 ounces each)

¼ cup panko bread crumbs

½ teaspoon salt-free
  mesquite seasoning

1 teaspoon olive oil

1 teaspoon butter

Healthy fish recipes are often baked or grilled, but who says you can't enjoy a flavorful crispy fillet that tastes as if you fried it? This inspired twist on fried fish is much lower in fat and higher in nutrients than a typical fish-and-chips meal. These also taste great made in an air fryer, if you have one (see tip).

1. In a small bowl, combine the mustard and sour cream. Spread the mustard mixture onto both sides of each salmon fillet, dividing evenly between the two.

2. Mix the panko bread crumbs and seasoning together in a small bowl. Press each fillet into the seasoned crumbs, lightly coating both sides.

3. Heat the oil and butter in a large nonstick skillet over medium-high heat. Place the fish into the hot fat to fry. Gently turn each fillet after 4 to 5 minutes, and pan-fry the other side for another 5 to 6 minutes until lightly browned. The salmon should change to a lighter color but not be opaque. Serve hot.

**COOKING TIP:** You can also air fry these fillets in an oven-style air fryer. Spray the breaded fillets with oil and bake them for 10 minutes at 400°F.

. . . . . . . . . . . . . . . . . . . . . . . . . . . . . . . . . . . . . . . . . . . . . . . . . . .

**Per Serving** Calories: 307; Total fat: 15g; Carbohydrates: 11g; Fiber: 1g; Protein: 31g; Calcium: 56mg; Sodium: 689mg; Potassium: 746mg; Vitamin D: 9mcg; Iron: 2mg; Zinc: 1mg

# Seared Ginger–Soy Ahi Tuna

✔ **30 MINUTES OR LESS**
✔ **ONE-POT**

**SERVES 2**

**PREP TIME:** 10 MINUTES
**COOK TIME:** 2 MINUTES

2 tablespoons reduced-
  sodium soy sauce, divided

Juice of 1 lime

2 teaspoons Dijon mustard

¼ teaspoon ground ginger

10 ounces sushi-grade tuna

1 teaspoon olive oil

4 scallions, both white and
  green parts, thinly sliced

The secret to great seared tuna at home is the type and freshness of the tuna. You want to use yellowfin sushi-grade tuna. You also don't want to overcook it. Source your tuna from a reputable fishmonger and ask about its quality. This dish can be enjoyed with a side of rice and sautéed or roasted vegetables.

1. In a small bowl, mix together 1 tablespoon of the soy sauce with the lime juice, mustard, and ginger until blended. Using a basting brush, brush the mixture onto each side of the tuna.

2. Heat the oil in a large nonstick skillet over high heat. Add the tuna, searing one side for 1 minute. Flip the fish over and sear the other side for 1 minute. The fish should still be pink in the middle.

3. Remove the tuna from the skillet, transfer it to a small serving platter, and cut it on the diagonal into ¼-inch slices. Top with the scallions and serve with the remaining soy sauce.

**SUBSTITUTION TIP:** You can use 1 teaspoon grated fresh ginger in place of the ground ginger.

. . . . . . . . . . . . . . . . . . . . . . . . . . . . . . . . . . . . . . . . . . . . . . . . . . .

**Per Serving** Calories: 126; Total fat: 5g; Carbohydrates: 3g; Fiber: 1g; Protein: 18g; Calcium: 22mg; Sodium: 313mg; Potassium: 263mg; Vitamin D: 4mcg; Iron: 1mg; Zinc: 1mg

# Greek-Style Cod with Olives & Tomatoes

✔ ONE-POT

**SERVES 2**

**PREP TIME:** 15 MINUTES
**COOK TIME:** 35 MINUTES

1 pint grape or cherry
  tomatoes, halved

⅓ cup mixed olives, pitted,
  roughly chopped

1 teaspoon olive oil

2 cod fillets
  (5 to 8 ounces each)

1 teaspoon Herbs
  de Provence

2 lemon wedges, for garnish

Cod lends itself well to this simple tomato-olive sauce. The olives in this dish add saltiness and flavor while keeping the overall sodium in check. Olives also provide those heart-healthy monounsaturated fats. Cooking down the tomatoes creates a rustic sauce for the fish. Serve this atop bow tie pasta or with a side of rice.

1. Preheat the oven to 375°F. Line a baking sheet with parchment paper or a silicone mat.

2. Place the tomatoes and olives on one half of the baking sheet and drizzle them with olive oil. Roast in the oven for 15 minutes.

3. Remove the baking sheet from the oven, place the cod fillets on the empty side, and season both the tomato mixture and the fish with Herbs de Provence. Bake for 15 to 20 minutes until the fish is opaque.

4. Serve the fish topped with the olive-tomato mixture and garnished with a squeeze of lemon.

**SUBSTITUTION TIP:** You can replace the cod with another whitefish.

. . . . . . . . . . . . . . . . . . . . . . . . . . . . . . . . . . . . . . . . . . . . . . . . . . . . . . .

**Per Serving** Calories: 186; Total fat: 6g; Carbohydrates: 8g; Fiber: 2g; Protein: 26g; Calcium: 53mg; Sodium: 244mg; Potassium: 813mg; Vitamin D: 1mcg; Iron: 2mg; Zinc: 1mg

# Pesto Tilapia

✔ **30 MINUTES OR LESS**
✔ **ONE-POT**

**SERVES 2**

**PREP TIME:** 5 MINUTES
**COOK TIME:** 20 MINUTES

¼ cup dry white wine

1 teaspoon avocado oil

1 lemon, halved

2 tilapia fillets
  (5 to 7 ounces each)

Freshly ground
  black pepper

2 tablespoons store-bought
  low-sodium pesto

The DASH diet encourages eating fish at least twice a week, and this flavor-packed recipe makes that easy. Fish is low in saturated fat and calories. Using a jarred pesto gets this delightful meal to the table even more quickly. When choosing a store-bought pesto, check the ingredients, and look for the brand with the lowest sodium.

1. Preheat the oven to 350°F.

2. In a 9-by-11-inch baking dish, whisk the wine, oil, and juice of half a lemon. Add the fish fillets and season lightly with pepper.

3. Cover the baking dish with foil and bake for 15 minutes. Uncover the dish, top each fillet with 1 tablespoon pesto, and cook for 5 more minutes.

4. Cut the remaining ½ lemon into wedges and serve each fillet with a lemon wedge.

**VARIATION TIP:** The pesto from the Sugar Snap Noodles with Gingered Pesto recipe (page 89) works great here—just omit the ginger if you'd like to make your own.

. . . . . . . . . . . . . . . . . . . . . . . . . . . . . . . . . . . . . . . . . . . . . . . . . . . . . . .

**Per Serving** Calories: 272; Total fat: 13g; Carbohydrates: 3g; Fiber: 0g; Protein: 30g; Calcium: 56mg; Sodium: 220mg; Potassium: 502mg; Vitamin D: 4mcg; Iron: 1mg; Zinc: 1mg

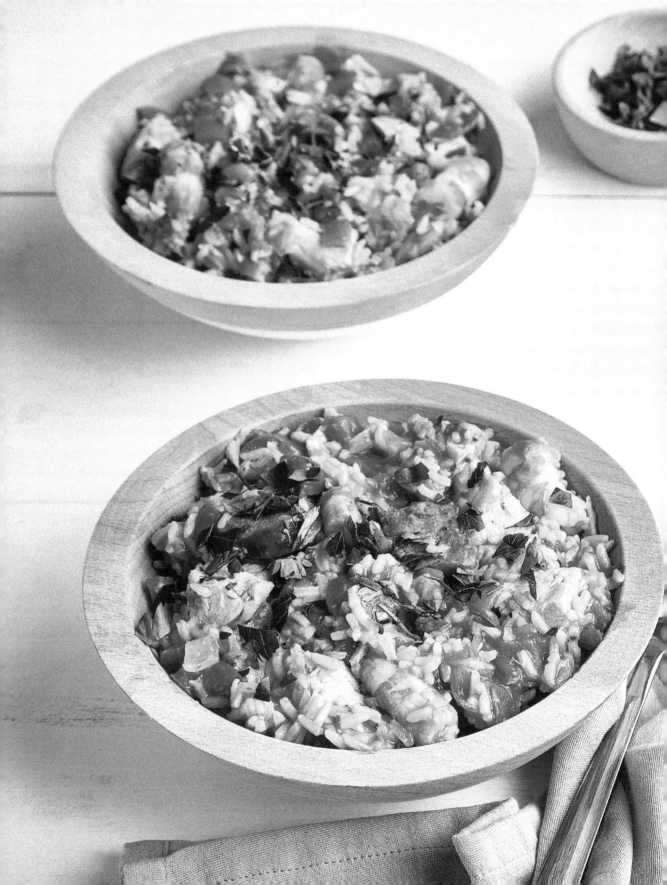

# 7
# POULTRY

# Buffalo Chicken Mac 'n' Cheese

**SERVES 4**

**PREP TIME:** 10 MINUTES
**COOK TIME:** 26 MINUTES

Nonstick cooking spray

½ cup chopped celery

1 tablespoon butter

1 tablespoon flour

2 cups 1 percent milk

¼ cup light cream cheese, cut into small cubes

2 tablespoons hot sauce (or to taste)

¼ teaspoon garlic powder

¼ teaspoon salt

¼ teaspoon freshly ground black pepper

½ cup shredded cheddar cheese

2 tablespoons blue cheese, crumbled

12 ounces roasted chicken breast, shredded

8 ounces elbow macaroni

Sometimes you just have a hankering for something indulgent. This dish has the flavors of Buffalo hot wings, without the extra fat and calories. Knowing how to make a basic white sauce allows you to enjoy decadent dishes while getting your DASH dairy servings. Enjoy this high-protein mac 'n' cheese with a side salad. Since it reheats well, this recipe provides 4 servings.

1. Fill a medium stockpot three-quarters full with water and bring it to a boil over high heat.

2. Lightly spray a large skillet with cooking spray and sauté the celery over medium heat until tender, about 3 to 4 minutes. Remove the celery from the skillet and set aside in a small bowl.

3. In the same skillet, melt the butter. Reduce the heat to medium-low and whisk in the flour until it's lightly browned, about 2 minutes.

4. Gradually add the milk, whisking for 2 minutes.

5. Add the cream cheese and continue to stir until melted, about 3 minutes. Add the hot sauce, garlic powder, salt, and pepper, and stir to combine.

6. Add the cheddar and blue cheese and stir to blend. Continue stirring until the sauce is smooth and thickened, about 3 minutes. Transfer the celery to the sauce. If the sauce is too thick, thin it with a little milk. Remove the sauce from the heat.

7. Add the cooked chicken to the sauce and stir until combined. Set the mixture aside or keep it warm over low heat.

8. Add the macaroni to the boiling water and cook for 8 to 9 minutes or until al dente.

9. Drain the macaroni and immediately add it to the chicken and sauce mixture, stirring to combine.

10. Transfer the pasta to 4 serving bowls and serve with additional hot sauce as desired.

**PREP TIP:** You can use an additional 1 to 2 tablespoons of light cream cheese to thicken the sauce.

. . . . . . . . . . . . . . . . . . . . . . . . . . . . . . . . . . . . . . . . . . . . . . . .

**Per Serving** Calories: 541; Total fat: 16g; Carbohydrates: 52g; Fiber: 2g; Protein: 44g; Calcium: 324mg; Sodium: 537mg; Potassium: 633mg; Vitamin D: 1mcg; Iron: 2mg; Zinc: 3mg

# Chicken & Fresh Veggie Tacos

✔ **30 MINUTES OR LESS**
✔ **ONE-POT**

**SERVES 2**

**PREP TIME:** 15 MINUTES
**COOK TIME:** 15 MINUTES

1 teaspoon avocado oil

1 bell pepper, diced

⅓ cup diced onion

1 (8- to 9-ounce) skinless, boneless chicken breast, cut into ¼-inch strips

¼ cup water

1 tablespoon low-sodium taco seasoning

1 lime, quartered

2 plum tomatoes, diced

1 tablespoon chopped cilantro, divided

4 corn taco shells

¼ cup nonfat Greek yogurt

Looking to use leftover chopped chicken? Look no further than this simple twist on traditional tacos. Using a salt-free or low-sodium taco seasoning reduces the sodium, and using chicken instead of beef lowers the saturated fat. Adding peppers, onions, and tomatoes works in a serving of fresh veggies. All those benefits and delicious as well!

1. Heat the oil in a large nonstick skillet over medium-high heat. Sauté the peppers and onions until tender, about 5 minutes. Transfer the veggies to a small bowl and return the skillet to the heat.

2. Add the chicken and sauté for 2 minutes. Add the water, taco seasoning, and the juice of half a lime. Reduce the heat to low, stirring to coat the chicken with the seasoning. Simmer for another 5 to 6 minutes over low heat, then remove from the heat and stir in the peppers and onions.

3. While the chicken simmers, in a small bowl stir together the tomatoes with 2 teaspoons cilantro. Heat the taco shells in the oven or toaster oven for 5 minutes.

4. Fill each taco with the chicken filling and the tomato mixture, and top each with 1 tablespoon of yogurt and the remaining cilantro.

5. Serve each person 2 tacos garnished with a lime wedge.

**INGREDIENT TIP:** You can make your own no-salt taco seasoning by blending 1 tablespoon chili powder, 1 teaspoon garlic powder, 1 teaspoon cumin, 1 teaspoon paprika, ¼ teaspoon cayenne pepper, and 1 teaspoon cornstarch.

. . . . . . . . . . . . . . . . . . . . . . . . . . . . . . . . . . . . . . . . . . . . . . . . . . .

**Per Serving** Calories: 346; Total fat: 11g; Carbohydrates: 30g; Fiber: 4g; Protein: 32g; Calcium: 88mg; Sodium: 150mg; Potassium: 888mg; Vitamin D: 0mcg; Iron: 2mg; Zinc: 2mg

# Sheet Pan Chicken Thighs

✔ BUDGET-SAVER

✔ ONE-POT

**SERVES 2**

**PREP TIME:** 20 MINUTES
**COOK TIME:** 35 MINUTES

4 skinless chicken thighs
(4 ounces each)

1 tablespoon mesquite
salt-free seasoning blend

1 teaspoon avocado oil

1 teaspoon Herbs
de Provence

Sheet pan dinners are incredibly simple to throw together with an assortment of proteins and heaps of vegetables. Chicken thighs are considered "dark meat," and while they're still relatively low in fat, they have a higher fat content than white meat. When you skip the skin, they're a great option with lots of flavor. Fill the rest of your plate with a salad or roasted veggies, such as the Garlicky Roasted Broccoli (page 163), and you'll have a fabulous and balanced quick dinner.

1. Heat the oven to 400°F. Line a baking sheet with parchment paper or a silicone mat.

2. Rub the chicken thighs with the seasoning blend and place them on the baking sheet. Drizzle the oil evenly over the thighs and sprinkle them with the herbs.

3. Bake the chicken for 35 minutes, or until cooked through, and serve.

**PREP TIP:** Add 1 cup of carrots and potatoes, cut into chunks, to the pan and roast them with the chicken to make this a complete meal.

. . . . . . . . . . . . . . . . . . . . . . . . . . . . . . . . . . . . . . . . . . . . . . . . . . . . . . .

**Per Serving** Calories: 294; Total fat: 12g; Carbohydrates: 0g; Fiber: 0g; Protein: 45g; Calcium: 16mg; Sodium: 215mg; Potassium: 549mg; Vitamin D: 0mcg; Iron: 2mg; Zinc: 4mg

# Chicken & Shrimp Jambalaya

✔ **BUDGET-SAVER**
✔ **ONE-POT**

**SERVES 2 TO 3**

**PREP TIME:** 20 MINUTES
**COOK TIME:** 30 MINUTES

1 teaspoon vegetable oil

2 bell peppers, diced

½ sweet onion, diced

½ teaspoon garlic powder

½ teaspoon onion powder

½ teaspoon paprika

¼ teaspoon
  cayenne pepper

¼ teaspoon oregano

1 (6- to 8-ounce) boneless,
  skinless chicken breast,
  cut into 1-inch chunks

1 (2.5-ounce) link andouille
  sausage, cut into 8 to
  10 pieces

2 cups no-salt-added
  chicken broth

1 cup chopped tomatoes

¾ cup long grain rice

6 shrimp, cooked, peeled,
  deveined, and tails off,
  coarsely chopped

2 tablespoons chopped
  parsley, for garnish

This one-pot jambalaya is a lower-fat, vegetable-heavy version of the original. The sausage is high in sodium but really adds to the flavor profile, so you'll use less of it and more chicken. The dish is prepared in one pan and uses frozen cooked shrimp to save time, but you can cook fresh shrimp if you prefer.

1. Heat the oil in a large nonstick skillet over medium heat. Add the peppers and onions. Cook until the vegetables are tender, about 3 to 4 minutes.

2. While the vegetables are cooking, in a small bowl mix together the garlic powder, onion powder, paprika, cayenne pepper, and oregano until well-blended.

3. Move the vegetables to the sides of the skillet and add the chicken in the empty space. Sprinkle the seasoning blend over the chicken and cook until it's opaque, 5 to 6 minutes.

4. Add the sausage, broth, tomatoes, and rice to the skillet and stir to combine.

5. Cover the skillet, reduce the heat to medium-low, and simmer for 10 to 12 minutes, until the liquid is almost absorbed. Stir in the shrimp. Cover again and simmer for an additional 5 minutes, or until all liquid is absorbed.

6. Serve in bowls, garnished with parsley.

**SUBSTITUTION TIP:** You can substitute 1½ tablespoons of salt-free Cajun seasoning for the garlic powder, onion powder, paprika, cayenne pepper, and oregano in the ingredient list.

**INGREDIENT TIP:** You can use 2 cups of frozen peppers and onions to save time.

**STORAGE TIP:** Store in an airtight container in the refrigerator for up to 3 days.

. . . . . . . . . . . . . . . . . . . . . . . . . . . . . . . . . . . . . . . . . . . . . . . . . . . . . . .

**Per Serving** Calories: 600; Total fat: 17g; Carbohydrates: 78g; Fiber: 7g; Protein: 35g; Calcium: 99mg; Sodium: 508mg; Potassium: 1218mg; Vitamin D: 0mcg; Iron: 4mg; Zinc: 3mg

# Quick Chicken Marsala

**SERVES 2**

**PREP TIME:** 15 MINUTES
**COOK TIME:** 25 MINUTES

1 (6-ounce) boneless
  skinless chicken breast,
  cut horizontally into
  2 pieces

¼ cup all-purpose flour

½ teaspoon salt-free
  Italian seasoning

2 teaspoons olive
  oil, divided

1 garlic clove, pressed
  or minced

2 cups sliced
  cremini mushrooms

6 ounces dry white wine

2 tablespoons
  chopped parsley

Zucchini noodles or
  cooked angel hair pasta,
  for serving

Plentiful mushrooms boost the nutrition in this classic recipe. Mushrooms are full of B vitamins and potassium. Cremini mushrooms, also known as "baby bellas," offer a little more depth to this lightened-up earthy dish. This recipe is another example of creating a meal for two with smaller portions of protein—in this case, chicken. Most chicken breasts are thick, but by cutting them horizontally, you can stretch one breast into a whole meal for two.

1. Place the chicken pieces between two pieces of wax paper. Using a meat mallet, pound until each piece is a little more than ¼-inch thick.

2. Mix together the flour and herb seasoning on a shallow plate. Dredge the chicken breast pieces in the seasoned flour and set aside.

3. Heat 1 teaspoon of oil in a large nonstick skillet over medium-high heat.

4. Add the chicken pieces and pan-fry, cooking each side for 3 to 5 minutes. Transfer the chicken to a plate and cover loosely with foil to keep warm.

5. Heat the remaining oil in the skillet and add the garlic and mushrooms. Cook for 5 to 6 minutes until the mushrooms are browned and their liquid has mostly evaporated. Add the wine to the skillet and simmer until it is slightly thickened, about 2 minutes.

6. Return the chicken back to the skillet and simmer for another 3 to 4 minutes.

7. Garnish with parsley and serve over zucchini noodles or angel hair pasta.

**SUBSTITUTION TIP:** You can substitute boneless, skinless chicken thighs for breasts. And if you can't find cremini mushrooms, standard white button mushrooms will do.

**STORAGE TIP:** Store in an airtight container in the refrigerator for up to 3 days.

. . . . . . . . . . . . . . . . . . . . . . . . . . . . . . . . . . . . . . . . . . . . . . . . . . . . . .

**Per Serving** Calories: 289; Total fat: 7g; Carbohydrates: 17g; Fiber: 1g; Protein: 23g; Calcium: 24mg; Sodium: 49mg; Potassium: 611mg; Vitamin D: 0mcg; Iron: 2mg; Zinc: 1mg

# Chicken Piccata with Vegetables

✓ ONE-POT

**SERVES 2**

**PREP TIME:** 15 MINUTES
**COOK TIME:** 23 MINUTES

1 (6-ounce) boneless
  skinless chicken breast,
  cut horizontally into
  two pieces

2 teaspoons olive
  oil, divided

1 red bell pepper, chopped

1 small green
  zucchini, sliced

1 small yellow
  zucchini, sliced

⅓ cup all-purpose flour

1 teaspoon dried oregano

6 ounces dry white wine

1 garlic clove, pressed
  or minced

1 small lemon, sliced

1 to 2 tablespoons chopped
  parsley, for garnish

This dish uses a similar method to the Quick Chicken Marsala
(page 122), but instead of mushrooms, lemons are the star.
To make this classic a better fit for DASH, I skipped the
high-sodium capers and added tender vegetables instead.
This dish pairs well with a small serving of linguine.

1. Place the chicken pieces between two pieces of wax
   paper. Using a meat mallet, pound until each piece is
   a little more than ¼-inch thick. Set aside.

2. Heat 1 teaspoon oil in a large nonstick skillet over
   medium-high heat. Add the peppers and cook for
   3 minutes or until tender. Add the green and yellow
   zucchini and sauté until crisp-tender, about 2 minutes.
   Remove from the heat and transfer to a small bowl.

3. Mix together the flour and oregano on a shallow plate.
   Dredge the chicken pieces in the seasoned flour.

4. Heat the remaining oil in the same skillet used for the
   vegetables over medium-high heat. Add the chicken and
   pan-fry it, cooking each side for 3 to 5 minutes.

5. Add the wine and garlic to the skillet and cook for 1 to
   2 minutes, allowing the liquid to reduce slightly. Add
   the vegetables and lemon slices to the skillet, reduce the
   heat to low, cover, and simmer for 2 to 3 minutes.

6. Serve garnished with parsley.

**STORAGE TIP:** Store in an airtight container in the refrigerator for up to 3 days.

. . . . . . . . . . . . . . . . . . . . . . . . . . . . . . . . . . . . . . . . . . . .

**Per Serving** Calories: 386; Total fat: 9g; Carbohydrates: 24g;
Fiber: 3g; Protein: 36g; Calcium: 55mg; Sodium: 82mg;
Potassium: 1032mg; Vitamin D: 0mcg; Iron: 3mg; Zinc: 2mg

# Ginger-Marinated Chicken Thighs

**SERVES 2**

**PREP TIME:** 10 MINUTES,
PLUS 1 HOUR TO MARINATE
**COOK TIME:** 14 MINUTES

2 tablespoons
 balsamic vinegar

2 teaspoons olive oil

2 teaspoons freshly
 grated ginger

1 garlic clove, pressed
 or minced

¼ teaspoon
 ground coriander

2 skinless chicken thighs
 (4 ounces each)

Nonstick cooking spray

Marinating chicken is one of the best methods to create an exciting blend of flavors like ginger, cilantro, and tangy balsamic vinegar. You can prepare this dish very quickly after the marinating time is complete, in less than 30 minutes of cooking time. Consider marinating the chicken early in the day, so it's ready to cook by dinnertime. Serve these thighs on a salad, or along with grilled asparagus and roasted potatoes.

1. Put the vinegar, oil, ginger, garlic, and coriander into a medium zip-top plastic bag, seal it, and shake the bag to combine the ingredients.

2. Add the chicken thighs to the bag, press out any excess air, and seal the bag. Marinate the chicken in the refrigerator for 1 hour or up to 10 hours.

3. Spray the grates of a grill with cooking spray and heat the grill to medium heat. Grill the chicken for about 5 to 7 minutes per side or until done, turning once. Discard the marinade.

4. If you do not have a grill, bake the chicken at 425°F in the oven for 35 minutes, turning once during baking, and serve.

**PREP TIP:** Consider doubling the recipe and grilling 4 thighs and freezing them for later use. You could slice them and have them ready to top a salad or go into another dish.

. . . . . . . . . . . . . . . . . . . . . . . . . . . . . . . . . . . . . . . . . . . . . .

**Per Serving** Calories: 196; Total fat: 9g; Carbohydrates: 4g; Fiber: 0g; Protein: 23g; Calcium: 15mg; Sodium: 112mg; Potassium: 307mg; Vitamin D: 0mcg; Iron: 1mg; Zinc: 2mg

# Peanut Chicken Stir-Fry

✔ **30 MINUTES OR LESS**
✔ **ONE-POT**

**SERVES 2**

**PREP TIME:** 15 MINUTES
**COOK TIME:** 15 MINUTES

3 tablespoons
  peanut butter

1 tablespoon reduced-
  sodium soy sauce

1 tablespoon canola or
  peanut oil, divided

6 ounces boneless, skinless
  chicken breast, cubed

1 bell pepper, cut into
  thin strips

½ sweet onion, cut into
  thin slices

1 cup broccoli florets

½ cup julienned carrots

⅓ cup chopped peanuts,
  plus 1 tablespoon

Cooked rice, for
  serving (optional)

2 tablespoons chopped
  scallions, for garnish

Stir-frying is an ancient Chinese cooking technique that uses high heat and a small amount of oil to produce healthy meals in record time. Veggies are often the star of stir-fries, and similar to this recipe, a small portion of meat goes a long way. Here I use carrots, bell peppers, and broccoli, but you can include a variety of vegetables.

1. In a small bowl, whisk together the peanut butter and soy sauce until blended. Set aside.

2. Heat 2 teaspoons of the oil in a nonstick wok or large nonstick skillet over high heat. Add the chicken and quickly stir-fry until there's no pink showing, about 5 minutes. Transfer the chicken to a small bowl and set aside.

3. Add the remaining oil to the wok or skillet and add the bell pepper, onion, broccoli, and carrots. Stir-fry until the broccoli and carrots are tender-crisp, about 3 minutes. Return the chicken to the skillet and stir-fry for 1 additional minute.

4. Add ⅓ cup chopped peanuts and the peanut butter–soy sauce mixture and toss to coat. Stir-fry for 2 more minutes.

5. Serve over rice (if using), garnished with scallions and the remaining 1 tablespoon chopped peanuts.

**SUBSTITUTION TIP:** You can substitute 6 ounces of lean beef or pork for the chicken. You can also substitute chopped cashews for the peanuts.

. . . . . . . . . . . . . . . . . . . . . . . . . . . . . . . . . . . . . . .

**Per Serving** Calories: 524; Total fat: 33g; Carbohydrates: 29g; Fiber: 7g; Protein: 34g; Calcium: 98mg; Sodium: 589mg; Potassium: 1079mg; Vitamin D: 0mcg; Iron: 3mg; Zinc: 3mg

# Chicken Breast with Yogurt Sauce & Chopped Walnuts

✓ **30 MINUTES OR LESS**
✓ **ONE-POT**

**SERVES 2 TO 3**

**PREP TIME:** 15 MINUTES
**COOK TIME:** 15 MINUTES

2 (5-ounce) boneless skinless chicken breasts, each
  cut into 3 pieces

½ teaspoon paprika

¼ teaspoon freshly ground
  black pepper

⅛ teaspoon salt

1 teaspoon avocado oil

¼ cup finely chopped onion

½ cup finely
  chopped walnuts

½ cup nonfat plain
  Greek yogurt

1 lemon, quartered

1 tablespoon chopped
  mint leaves

This light meal is a fusion of classic Hungarian and Middle Eastern dishes, combining chicken, paprika, yogurt, walnuts, and mint into something sublime. The walnuts add some omega-3 fatty acids and protein. Pair this with a side of rice pilaf or serve it over steamed vegetable noodles.

1. Season the chicken on all sides with the paprika, pepper, and salt.

2. Heat the oil in a large nonstick skillet over medium heat. Add the chicken pieces and cook for 3 to 4 minutes per side. Add the onion to the skillet and stir. Continue cooking until the chicken is no longer pink and the onion is translucent, about 5 minutes. Remove from the heat.

3. Put the walnuts, yogurt, juice of half the lemon, and mint in a food processor and pulse until well-blended and smooth.

4. Serve the chicken with the yogurt sauce and garnished with the lemon wedges.

**SUBSTITUTION TIP:** You can substitute basil or parsley for the mint if you prefer.

**STORAGE TIP:** Store in an airtight container in the refrigerator for up to 3 days.

**Per Serving** Calories: 430; Total fat: 25g; Carbohydrates: 10g; Fiber: 3g; Protein: 42g; Calcium: 106mg; Sodium: 241mg; Potassium: 750mg; Vitamin D: 0mcg; Iron: 2mg; Zinc: 2mg

# Creamy Chicken Breast with Spinach & Mushrooms

✔ **30 MINUTES OR LESS**
✔ **ONE-POT**

**SERVES 2 TO 3**

**PREP TIME:** 10 MINUTES
**COOK TIME:** 20 MINUTES

½ teaspoon olive oil

2 (5-ounce) boneless, skinless chicken breasts, cubed

8 ounces sliced mushrooms

¼ cup chopped onion

2 teaspoons unsalted butter

1 tablespoon all-purpose flour

1 cup 1 percent milk

2 tablespoons light cream cheese

¼ cup shredded Swiss or Gruyère cheese

1 (10-ounce) bag fresh baby spinach, chopped

This recipe is a spin on the retro comfort-food dish Chicken à la King. It's creamy and delicious but lower in saturated fat than the original. Spinach and extra mushrooms give this a nutrition boost. If you want to mimic the flashback dish, stir in ½ cup of chopped roasted red pepper.

1. In a medium saucepan, heat the oil over medium-high heat and sauté the chicken for 3 to 4 minutes. Add the mushrooms and onions, stir to combine, and cover. Reduce the heat to low and simmer for 5 to 6 minutes. Transfer the mixture to a small bowl.

2. Melt the butter over medium heat in the same saucepan. Whisk in the flour for 1 minute. Slowly pour in the milk, whisking, and bring it to a boil. Reduce the heat to low, and while the sauce is simmering, stir in the cream cheese and the shredded cheese and continue stirring until the sauce is creamy and well blended, about 3 minutes.

3. Return the chicken and mushroom mixture to the sauce. Add the spinach, stir, and cook over low heat for 2 to 3 minutes until the spinach is wilted and the chicken is heated through.

4. Serve over rice or your favorite cooked grain.

**STORAGE TIP:** Store in an airtight container in the refrigerator for up to 3 days.

· · · · · · · · · · · · · · · · · · · · · · · · · · · · · · · · · · · · · · · · · · · · · · · · · · · · · · · ·

**Per Serving** Calories: 424; Total fat: 16g; Carbohydrates: 22g; Fiber: 6g; Protein: 50g; Calcium: 519mg; Sodium: 388mg; Potassium: 1374mg; Vitamin D: 2mcg; Iron: 5mg; Zinc: 4mg

# Cheesy Chicken Pizza with Chili Oil & Pineapple

✔ 30 MINUTES OR LESS
✔ ONE-POT

**SERVES 2**

**PREP TIME:** 10 MINUTES
**COOK TIME:** 15 MINUTES

2 teaspoons olive oil, divided

3 ounces skinless, boneless chicken breast, thinly sliced

2 pieces naan, or another flatbread

2 plum tomatoes, chopped

3 ounces fresh mozzarella, thinly sliced

1 (8-ounce) can crushed pineapple, drained

1 teaspoon hot chili oil

½ teaspoon honey

Who doesn't like pizza? Even though naan contains a bit of sodium, using it for the crust brings this dish together in minutes. Choosing fresh mozzarella over the packaged part-skim shredded type helps lower the sodium count. Making a quick pizza at home can satisfy your craving while reducing sodium and fat significantly (compared to pizzeria pies).

1. Preheat the oven to 400°F.

2. Heat 1 teaspoon of olive oil in a small nonstick skillet over medium-high heat and sauté the chicken until cooked through, about 6 to 7 minutes.

3. Drizzle the remaining oil onto the naan. Top each piece evenly with the chopped tomatoes and sliced chicken.

4. Add the slices of mozzarella and the pineapple. Drizzle both pizzas evenly with chili oil and honey.

5. Bake for 8 minutes on a pizza stone, or directly on the oven rack, until lightly browned and crisp. Serve.

**SUBSTITUTION TIP:** You can use mini pizza flatbread crusts if you can't find naan. Just make sure to check the labels for fat and sodium.

. . . . . . . . . . . . . . . . . . . . . . . . . . . . . . . . . . . . . . . . . . . . . . . . . . . .

**Per Serving** Calories: 585; Total fat: 23g; Carbohydrates: 68g; Fiber: 4g; Protein: 29g; Calcium: 317mg; Sodium: 709mg; Potassium: 575mg; Vitamin D: 0mcg; Iron: 4mg; Zinc: 2mg

# Greek Sheet Pan Chicken

**SERVES 2**

**PREP TIME:** 10 MINUTES
**COOK TIME:** 45 MINUTES

2 boneless, skinless chicken
  breasts (5 ounces each)

1 cup grape
  tomatoes, halved

1 small zucchini, sliced

½ cup chopped onions

⅓ cup chopped, pitted
  mixed olives, packed in oil

1 teaspoon salt-free
  Greek seasoning

Freshly ground
  black pepper

1 teaspoon olive
  oil (optional)

¼ cup feta cheese crumbles

This flavorful dish is high in healthy monounsaturated
fat and counts for two servings of vegetables. The prep is
simple and done on a single baking sheet, so clean up is a
breeze, too. You can purchase mixed olives in a jar and have
extra, or just buy what you need at a grocery store olive bar.
You'll need about a teaspoon of the oil from the olives to
create the vegetable topping.

1. Preheat the oven to 400°F. Line a baking sheet with
   parchment paper or a silicone mat.

2. Place the chicken breasts on the baking sheet
   (cut them in half horizontally if they are more than
   an inch thick).

3. In a small bowl, mix together the tomatoes, zucchini,
   onions, olives, and seasoning. Season to taste with
   pepper and toss. If the olives didn't have enough oil in
   them, add a teaspoon of olive oil. Top the chicken pieces
   with the tomato and olive mixture.

4. Cover the baking sheet loosely with foil and bake for
   25 minutes. Remove the foil and bake for another
   10 minutes. Top the chicken with the feta cheese and
   return it to the oven for 5 to 7 more minutes. Serve hot.

**SUBSTITUTION TIP:** Replace the Greek seasoning with individual dried herbs: ¼ teaspoon garlic powder, ½ teaspoon
oregano, and ¼ teaspoon parsley.

**STORAGE TIP:** Store wrapped in foil in the refrigerator for
up to 3 days.

. . . . . . . . . . . . . . . . . . . . . . . . . . . . . . . . . . . . . . . . . . . .

**Per Serving** Calories: 276; Total fat: 9g; Carbohydrates: 12g;
Fiber: 3g; Protein: 37g; Calcium: 160mg; Sodium: 421mg;
Potassium: 861mg; Vitamin D: 0mcg; Iron: 3mg; Zinc: 2mg

# Air-Fried Turkey Cutlets

✔ 30 MINUTES OR LESS
✔ ONE-POT

**SERVES 2**

**PREP TIME:** 15 MINUTES
**COOK TIME:** 10 MINUTES

Nonstick cooking spray

3 tablespoons
 all-purpose flour

1 large egg

⅓ cup bread crumbs

½ teaspoon dried oregano

¼ teaspoon garlic powder

8 ounces turkey
 breast cutlets

These homemade cutlets are a real treat. Serve them on top of a mixed green salad or eat them as is with a side of veggies. You can also eat them schnitzel-style, alongside Noodles with Mushrooms & Cabbage (page 87). If you don't have an air fryer, see the tip for conventional oven directions.

1. Preheat an oven-style air fryer to 400°F. Spray a small baking sheet with cooking spray and set aside.

2. Put the flour on a shallow plate. Crack the egg into a small bowl and beat it until blended. Mix the bread crumbs, oregano, and garlic powder together on another shallow plate.

3. Dredge each cutlet in the flour, then the egg, then the bread crumbs.

4. Place the breaded cutlets on the prepared baking sheet and spray the cutlets with cooking spray.

5. Bake on the air fry setting for 9 minutes. Serve hot.

**VARIATION TIP:** If you don't have an oven-style air fryer, use a conventional oven set to 425°F and bake for 20 minutes.

. . . . . . . . . . . . . . . . . . . . . . . . . . . . . . . . . . . . . . . . . . . . . .

**Per Serving** Calories: 281; Total fat: 6g; Carbohydrates: 22g; Fiber: 1g; Protein: 33g; Calcium: 63mg; Sodium: 250mg; Potassium: 393mg; Vitamin D: 0mcg; Iron: 3mg; Zinc: 2mg

# Turkey and Broccoli Alfredo

✓ ONE-POT

**SERVES 2**

**PREP TIME:** 10 MINUTES
**COOK TIME:** 25 MINUTES

½ teaspoon olive oil

8 ounces turkey breast
  cutlets, cut into thin strips

2 teaspoons
  unsalted butter

1 tablespoon
  all-purpose flour

1 cup 1 percent milk

2 tablespoons light
  cream cheese

¼ cup grated
  Parmesan cheese

4 ounces fettuccine

2 cups broccoli florets

Alfredo sauce is one of the most luscious sauces, synonymous with butter, cream, and heaps of fat-laden cheese. So, it is delightful that this delicious alfredo dish provides two servings of vegetables and is not a diet-busting meal. You can substitute vegetable noodles for the pasta if you really want to up your veggie count. The turkey cutlets provide lean protein, zinc, phosphorous, iron, and B vitamins.

1. Fill a large stockpot three-quarters full with water and bring it to a boil over high heat.

2. Heat the oil in a large nonstick skillet over medium-high heat. Add the turkey and sauté for 4 to 5 minutes until it is no longer pink. Transfer the turkey to a bowl, cover it with foil, and set aside.

3. Melt the butter in the same skillet over medium heat. Whisk in the flour for 1 minute. Slowly pour in the milk and bring to boil. Reduce the heat to low and, while simmering, stir in the cream cheese until it melts, about 3 minutes. Add the Parmesan cheese and continue stirring until the sauce is creamy and well-blended, about 3 minutes. Remove the sauce from the heat, transfer the cooked turkey to the sauce, and cover the pan to keep it warm.

4. Add the fettuccine to the boiling water and cook for 6 minutes. Add the broccoli and boil for 3 minutes more. Drain the pasta and broccoli, then transfer to a serving bowl.

5. Pour the sauce over the pasta and broccoli, gently toss, and serve.

**SUBSTITUTION TIP:** You can use cooked chicken in place of turkey. You can also use whole-wheat pasta or vegetable pasta in place of the fettucine.

**STORAGE TIP:** Store in an airtight container in the refrigerator for up to 3 days.

. . . . . . . . . . . . . . . . . . . . . . . . . . . . . . . . . . . . . . . . . . . . . . . . . . .

**Per Serving** Calories: 563; Total fat: 16g; Carbohydrates: 60g; Fiber: 4g; Protein: 46g; Calcium: 348mg; Sodium: 451mg; Potassium: 965mg; Vitamin D: 1mcg; Iron: 4mg; Zinc: 4mg

# Turkey and Spinach Stuffed Shells

✔ **MAKE-AHEAD**

**SERVES 2 TO 3**

**PREP TIME:** 20 MINUTES
**COOK TIME:** 55 MINUTES

⅛ teaspoon salt

Nonstick cooking spray

1 (8-ounce) bag fresh baby
  spinach, chopped

8 jumbo pasta shells

½ teaspoon olive oil

¼ cup minced onion

1 garlic clove, pressed
  or minced

8 ounces lean
  ground turkey

1½ cups part-skim
  ricotta cheese

1 cup shredded part-skim
  mozzarella cheese, divided

2 tablespoons minced
  fresh parsley

Pinch freshly ground
  black pepper

1½ cups tomato
  sauce, divided

This is a lovely dish to double up or make for company because it freezes and reheats well and is spectacular. To round out the meal, serve it with a large green salad. To reduce the sodium, make your own tomato sauce using no-salt-added canned tomato purée or diced tomatoes.

1. Fill a large stockpot three-quarters full with water, add the salt, and bring it to a boil over high heat.

2. Preheat the oven to 375°F. Spray a 9-by-11-inch baking dish with cooking spray.

3. Bring a half cup of water to a simmer in a large skillet over medium-high heat. Once it's simmering, add the spinach, cover, and steam for 2 to 3 minutes. Drain off any leftover water, and transfer the spinach to a small bowl.

4. Cook the shells in the boiling water for 8 minutes, then carefully drain and transfer them to a baking sheet.

5. While the shells cook, heat the oil in the same skillet used for the spinach. Add the onion and sauté for 2 minutes. Add the garlic and sauté for 1 minute. Add the ground turkey and cook for 6 to 8 minutes or until it is no longer pink, stirring occasionally. Remove the skillet from the heat.

6. In a medium bowl, mix together the ricotta, all but 2 tablespoons of the mozzarella, and the parsley and pepper until well combined. Fold in the spinach and cooked turkey.

7. Add ½ cup of tomato sauce to the bottom of the prepared baking dish.

**8.** Stuff each shell with the turkey-ricotta mixture and place the stuffed shells in the baking dish, open side up. Top each shell with the remaining tomato sauce and sprinkle evenly with the remaining mozzarella. Cover the dish with foil and bake for 25 minutes. Uncover, continue baking for 5 more minutes, and serve.

**STORAGE TIP:** You can freeze this dish for up to 3 months. Consider freezing in individual portions, then defrost in the refrigerator or microwave and bake as directed.

. . . . . . . . . . . . . . . . . . . . . . . . . . . . . . . . . . . . . . . . . . . . . . . . . . . . .

**Per Serving** Calories: 907; Total fat: 39g; Carbohydrates: 73g; Fiber: 8g; Protein: 70g; Calcium: 1131mg; Sodium: 714mg; Potassium: 1542mg; Vitamin D: 1mcg; Iron: 8mg; Zinc: 9mg

# Herbed Roast Turkey Breast

✔ ONE-POT

**SERVES 4**

**PREP TIME:** 10 MINUTES
**COOK TIME:** 45 MINUTES

1 teaspoon olive oil

1 (2-pound) split
  turkey breast

1 teaspoon salt-free Greek
  seasoning blend

⅛ teaspoon salt

Depending on the size of the turkey breast, you'll get at least four meals out of this recipe. You can use the cooked turkey in other meals, like the Turkey and Broccoli Alfredo (page 132), or you can make thick, satisfying sandwiches with the leftovers. Look for a fresh turkey breast that's been split by the store butcher. You can usually find a split breast that's around 1½ pounds. Check the package, however, because some poultry products have injected sodium.

1. Preheat the oven to 375°F.

2. Rub the oil all over the turkey breast, then rub in the seasoning and salt. Transfer the breast to a baking sheet and cover it loosely with foil.

3. Roast the turkey in the oven for 35 minutes. Remove the foil and roast for 10 more minutes.

4. Remove the turkey from the oven and let it rest for 5 to 10 minutes. Carve it into slices and serve.

**PREP TIP:** Omit the salt if the brand of turkey you purchased has salt added. If the turkey has the skin on, you can rub the herbs under skin and roast it. Remove the skin before eating.

**STORAGE TIP:** Store in an airtight container in the refrigerator for up to 3 days, or freeze leftovers for up to 3 months.

. . . . . . . . . . . . . . . . . . . . . . . . . . . . . . . . . . . . . . . . . . . . . . . . . . .

**Per Serving** Calories: 268; Total fat: 6g; Carbohydrates: 0g; Fiber: 0g; Protein: 53g; Calcium: 20mg; Sodium: 245mg; Potassium: 606mg; Vitamin D: 0mcg; Iron: 2mg; Zinc: 3mg

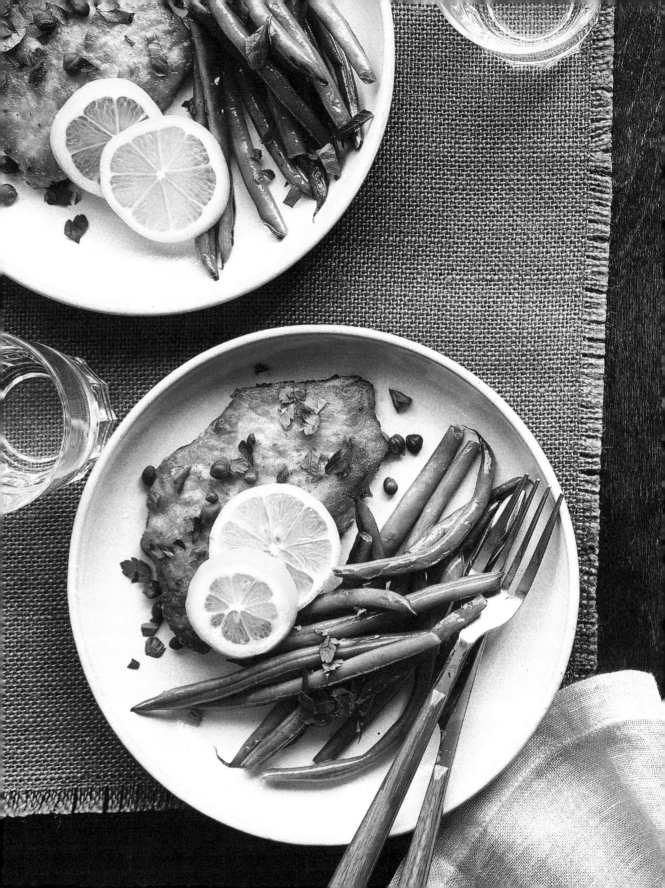

# 8

# PORK AND BEEF

# Pork Quinoa Bowls with Avocado, Peppers & Tomatoes

✔ **30 MINUTES OR LESS**
✔ **BUDGET-SAVER**
✔ **ONE-POT**

**SERVES 2**

**PREP TIME:** 5 MINUTES
**COOK TIME:** 20 MINUTES

1 teaspoon avocado
 oil, divided

¾ cup quinoa, rinsed

1⅓ cups low-sodium
 vegetable broth

1 large yellow bell
 pepper, diced

⅓ cup diced sweet onion

6 ounces ground pork

1 garlic clove, pressed
 or minced

½ teaspoon
 smoked paprika

¼ teaspoon
 cayenne pepper

1 tablespoon
 reduced-sodium soy sauce

2 tablespoons water

1 tablespoon brown sugar

1½ cups chopped tomatoes

1 avocado, sliced

Cilantro, for
 garnish (optional)

Bowls have become more popular of late, and for good reason. They combine multiple textures and flavors in one bowl and are usually packed with vegetables. This bowl uses quinoa instead of rice, which adds fiber and protein to balance out the smaller portion of pork. If possible, have your butcher grind pork loin for you. Ground pork is higher in fat than other types of meat, but this recipe uses a small amount of it.

1. Heat ½ teaspoon of oil in a large saucepan over medium heat. Add the quinoa and toast for 1 minute. Add the broth and bring to a boil. Once the broth is boiling, reduce the heat to low, cover, and cook for 10 minutes. Remove the saucepan from the heat and keep covered for 5 minutes. Fluff the quinoa with a fork and set aside.

2. While the quinoa cooks, heat the remaining ½ teaspoon of oil over medium heat in a small nonstick skillet. Add the peppers and onions and sauté until tender, about 3 to 4 minutes. Transfer the veggies to a bowl.

3. Add the ground pork to the same skillet, along with the garlic, paprika, and cayenne pepper. Cook the pork over medium heat for 5 to 6 minutes until lightly browned. Drain off any fat, then cook an additional 1 to 2 minutes until slightly caramelized. Remove the skillet from the heat.

4. In a small bowl, mix together the soy sauce, water, and brown sugar.

5. Divide the quinoa evenly between two small serving bowls. Place half of the ground pork over the quinoa down the middle of each bowl, half of the tomatoes and half of the avocado slices on the left side of the bowl, and half of the pepper mixture on the right side. Drizzle both bowls with the soy glaze, dividing it evenly, and garnish them with the cilantro, if using.

**VARIATION TIP:** Instead of using ground pork, you could slow-roast a whole pork loin, shred part of it for this dish, and freeze the rest for future meals.

. . . . . . . . . . . . . . . . . . . . . . . . . . . . . . . . . . . . . . . . . . . . . . . . . . . . . . . . .

**Per Serving** Calories: 751; Total fat: 40g; Carbohydrates: 72g; Fiber: 16g; Protein: 30g; Calcium: 99mg; Sodium: 255mg; Potassium: 1407mg; Vitamin D: 0mcg; Iron: 5mg; Zinc: 5mg

# Pork Tenderloin Medallions with Dijon–Yogurt Sauce

✔ **30 MINUTES OR LESS**
✔ **MAKE-AHEAD**
✔ **ONE-POT**

**SERVES 3**

**PREP TIME:** 10 MINUTES
**COOK TIME:** 10 MINUTES

1 teaspoon paprika

1 teaspoon dried oregano

½ teaspoon garlic powder

¼ teaspoon salt

1 teaspoon olive oil

1 (1-to-1¼ pound) pork tenderloin

¾ cup plain nonfat Greek yogurt

1 teaspoon Dijon mustard

1 teaspoon prepared barbecue sauce

These appetizing pork medallions are easy enough for every day but so delicious that they're also worthy of a special occasion. Be sure to buy a plain pork tenderloin, not one that has already been seasoned. This dish can be made ahead by prepping the tenderloin and then refrigerating it until you're ready to cook. Serve this with your favorite veggie or with the Bibb Lettuce with Beets, Pears & Goat Cheese on page 36.

1. In a small bowl, stir together the paprika, oregano, garlic powder, and salt until well blended.

2. Cut the meat into 12 slices, each a little over ½ inch thick. Rub each slice with a bit of the spice mixture.

3. Heat the oil in a large oven-safe skillet over medium heat. Place the pork tenderloin slices into the skillet and cook for 4 to 5 minutes per side, turning once. Cover and continue to cook over low heat for an additional 5 to 6 minutes.

4. While the medallions finish cooking, mix together the yogurt, mustard, and barbecue sauce in a small bowl.

5. Plate the pork in servings of 4 slices each, drizzle the sauce over the medallions, and serve.

**STORAGE TIP:** Store in an airtight container in the refrigerator for up to 3 days.

. . . . . . . . . . . . . . . . . . . . . . . . . . . . . . . . . . . . . . . . . . . . . . . . . .

**Per Serving** Calories: 207; Total fat: 4g; Carbohydrates: 4g; Fiber: 1g; Protein: 38g; Calcium: 79mg; Sodium: 334mg; Potassium: 718mg; Vitamin D: 0mcg; Iron: 2mg; Zinc: 3mg

# Pork Loin with Apples

✔ **30 MINUTES OR LESS**

✔ **ONE-POT**

**SERVES 2**

**PREP TIME:** 10 MINUTES
**COOK TIME:** 15 MINUTES

1 teaspoon ground thyme

½ teaspoon ground sage

1 teaspoon cinnamon, divided

¼ teaspoon salt

2 (3-ounce) boneless pork loin chops

½ teaspoon olive oil

½ cup thinly sliced red onion

2 Fuji apples, peeled, cored and sliced

¼ teaspoon nutmeg

Gone are the days of overcooking pork. The USDA recommends cooking pork chops, loin, and roasts to a temperature of 145°F for medium-rare, followed by a 3-minute rest. For medium, cook to 150°F to 155°F; for medium-well, it's 160°F. This quick, fuss-free meal also includes a serving of fruit. And although I use Fujis for their sweetness and firmness, you can use any variety of apples you prefer.

1. In a small bowl, mix together the thyme, sage, ½ teaspoon of the cinnamon, and salt. Rub each chop with the mixture.

2. Heat the oil in a large nonstick skillet over medium heat. Add the pork chops and onions to the skillet. Sear the chops for 1 minute per side, then cover. Cook for 2 minutes. Remove the lid and push the onions and pork to one side of the skillet.

3. Add the apples to the other side of the skillet and sprinkle them evenly with the remaining cinnamon and the nutmeg. If necessary, add a little water to the skillet. Cover the skillet, reduce the heat to low, cook for 5 to 6 minutes until the apples are tender, and serve.

**SUBSTITUTION TIP:** Unsweetened spiced applesauce can stand in for the sautéed apples if you are short on time or ingredients.

**STORAGE TIP:** Store in an airtight container in the refrigerator for up to 3 days.

. . . . . . . . . . . . . . . . . . . . . . . . . . . . . . . . . . . . . . . . . . . . . . . . . .

**Per Serving** Calories: 213; Total fat: 4g; Carbohydrates: 25g; Fiber: 4g; Protein: 20g; Calcium: 38mg; Sodium: 334mg; Potassium: 527mg; Vitamin D: 0mcg; Iron: 1mg; Zinc: 2mg

# Pork Stir-Fry

✔ **30 MINUTES OR LESS**
✔ **BUDGET-SAVER**
✔ **ONE-POT**

**SERVES 2**

**PREP TIME:** 10 MINUTES
**COOK TIME:** 10 MINUTES

2 teaspoons canola oil, divided

4 ounces boneless pork loin, thinly sliced

1 bell pepper, thinly sliced

½ cup sliced onion

1 cup packaged cabbage slaw

1 tablespoon reduced-sodium soy sauce

1 teaspoon honey

If you're looking for a budget-friendly meal that's packed with flavor and texture, stir-fries fit the bill perfectly. Using pre-shredded cabbage helps you get this dish to the table quickly, making it a stellar choice for hectic weeknights. You can easily double the portion if you'd like to invite the neighbors over or want a tasty lunch the following day.

1. Heat 1 teaspoon of oil in a wok or large nonstick skillet over medium-high heat. Add the pork and stir-fry for 3 to 4 minutes. Transfer the meat to a small bowl.

2. Heat the remaining teaspoon of oil in the wok, then add the pepper, onion, and cabbage. Stir-fry for 2 to 3 minutes. Return the pork to the skillet and toss all to combine. Add the soy sauce and honey to the mixture and stir-fry for another 2 minutes.

3. Serve over rice or your favorite cooked grain.

**INGREDIENT TIP:** You can add just about any vegetables to this dish. Try mushrooms and zucchini if you don't have cabbage on hand.

**STORAGE TIP:** Store in an airtight container in the refrigerator for up to 3 days.

. . . . . . . . . . . . . . . . . . . . . . . . . . . . . . . . . . . . . . . . . . . . . . . . . .

**Per Serving** Calories: 173; Total fat: 7g; Carbohydrates: 13g; Fiber: 3g; Protein: 15g; Calcium: 36mg; Sodium: 299mg; Potassium: 515mg; Vitamin D: 0mcg; Iron: 1mg; Zinc: 1mg

# Lemon Caper Pork Cutlets

✔ 30 MINUTES OR LESS

✔ BUDGET-SAVER

✔ ONE-POT

**SERVES 2**

**PREP TIME:** 15 MINUTES

**COOK TIME:** 10 MINUTES

2 (3-ounce) boneless pork cutlets

Pinch salt

½ teaspoon canola oil

¼ cup all-purpose flour

⅓ cup white wine

1 teaspoon capers

1 lemon, sliced

1 tablespoon chopped parsley, for garnish

Lemon and capers are traditionally combined in many dishes because their flavors play so well off each other. Brined capers are salty and lemons are sour, so the duo wakes up two taste areas on your tongue. A 3-ounce boneless pork cutlet contains less than 2 grams of saturated fat, so it fits nicely into a DASH plan. Surround the golden cutlets with lots of vegetables to complete your balanced meal.

1. Place the cutlets, one at a time, between two sheets of wax paper. Using a meat mallet, pound each cutlet to about ¼ inch in thickness. Lightly salt the cutlets.

2. Heat the oil in a medium nonstick skillet over medium-high heat.

3. Put the flour on a small plate and dredge the cutlets in it before placing them into the skillet. Cook for 2 minutes per side.

4. Add the wine, capers, and lemon slices (reserving 2 for garnish) to the skillet. Reduce the heat, cover, and simmer for 5 to 6 minutes.

5. Serve garnished with parsley and the reserved lemon slices.

**PREP TIP:** You can pound and prepare the cutlets, then refrigerate them until ready to cook.

**STORAGE TIP:** Store in an airtight container in the refrigerator for up to 3 days.

**Per Serving** Calories: 218; Total fat: 5g; Carbohydrates: 15g; Fiber: 1g; Protein: 21g; Calcium: 11mg; Sodium: 154mg; Potassium: 371mg; Vitamin D: 0mcg; Iron: 1mg; Zinc: 2mg

# Veal Marsala

✔ 30 MINUTES OR LESS
✔ ONE-POT

**SERVES 2**

**PREP TIME:** 15 MINUTES
**COOK TIME:** 10 MINUTES

8 ounces veal cutlets

⅛ teaspoon salt

Pinch freshly ground
 black pepper

3 tablespoons all-purpose
 flour, divided

1 teaspoon olive oil

1½ cups sliced mushrooms

1 cup diced bell peppers

¼ cup diced onion

2 garlic cloves, pressed
 or minced

½ cup dry white wine

½ cup low-sodium
 chicken broth

This is a classic Italian dish that I've DASH-ed up by adding more vegetables and using a smaller amount of veal. You can easily substitute boneless pork loin chops for the veal if you prefer. Pair this with the Roasted Potato Party (page 173) and a Caprese Tomato Salad (page 38).

1. Place the veal between two pieces of wax paper and pound with a mallet to ¼-inch thickness.

2. Season both sides of the meat with salt and pepper. Place 2 tablespoons of flour in a shallow dish and dredge the cutlets in it, one at a time.

3. Heat the oil over medium heat in a large nonstick skillet. Cook the cutlets for 2 minutes per side, turning once, until lightly browned. Transfer the cutlets to a small dish and set aside.

4. In the same skillet, sauté the mushrooms, peppers, onions, and garlic for 2 to 3 minutes, then add the wine. Cook for another 2 minutes and reduce the heat to low.

5. In a small bowl or glass measuring cup, mix the remaining tablespoon of flour with the broth and stir until blended. Gradually pour the broth into the skillet with the mushroom mixture and stir for 1 to 2 minutes or until slightly thickened.

6. Return the veal to the skillet and heat through for another 1 to 2 minutes, then serve immediately.

**SUBSTITUTION TIP:** You can use low-sodium vegetable broth or white wine in place of the chicken broth.

· · · · · · · · · · · · · · · · · · · · · · · · · · · · · · · · · · · · · · · · · · · · · · · · · ·

**Per Serving** Calories: 271; Total fat: 6g; Carbohydrates: 17g; Fiber: 2g; Protein: 28g; Calcium: 29mg; Sodium: 273mg; Potassium: 532mg; Vitamin D: 1mcg; Iron: 2mg; Zinc: 3mg

# Skillet Meatballs

**SERVES 2 TO 3**

**PREP TIME:** 15 MINUTES
**COOK TIME:** 15 MINUTES

**For the Meatballs**

6 ounces 90 percent lean ground beef

2 ounces lean ground turkey

½ cup plain bread crumbs

1 large egg

2 tablespoons milk

2 teaspoons minced fresh parsley or ½ teaspoon dried

⅛ teaspoon salt

Pinch freshly ground black pepper

Nonstick cooking spray

**For the Sauce**

½ teaspoon olive oil

1 garlic clove, pressed or minced

1 (14-ounce) can diced tomatoes

¼ teaspoon red pepper flakes (optional)

3 ounces fresh mozzarella cheese

This is another one-pan meal that is a lifesaver when your day is packed with activities. These lean meatballs can be enjoyed with a side salad and crusty whole-grain bread. You can use 8 ounces of turkey instead of a beef-turkey mixture if you'd prefer. Top a heaping plate of zucchini noodles with the rich sauce and tender meatballs for a comforting meal.

**To Make the Meatballs**

1. Place the beef, turkey, bread crumbs, egg, milk, parsley, salt, and pepper in a large bowl. Mix until all of the ingredients are well blended, then form the mixture into 8 meatballs.

2. Heat a large nonstick skillet over medium-high heat. Spray with cooking spray and add the meatballs. Cook for 6 to 7 minutes, turning gently so that each side browns. Transfer the meatballs to a plate and set them aside.

**To Make the Sauce**

3. Add the olive oil and garlic to the same skillet. Cook for 1 minute until the garlic is lightly browned. Add the tomatoes and red pepper flakes (if using). Transfer the meatballs back to the skillet and cook them with the sauce over medium heat until it just begins to boil. Cover, reduce the heat to low, and simmer for 5 more minutes.

4. Cut the mozzarella cheese into small chunks. Uncover the sauce and spread the cheese over the top. Replace the lid, simmer for another 2 minutes until the cheese melts, and serve.

CONTINUED ▶

**PREP TIP:** To brown the cheese, you can place the skillet beneath a preheated broiler for 1 minute in step 4.

**STORAGE TIP:** Store in an airtight container in the refrigerator for up to 3 days.

. . . . . . . . . . . . . . . . . . . . . . . . . . . . . . . . . . . . . . . . . . . . . . . . . . .

**Per Serving** Calories: 516; Total fat: 26g; Carbohydrates: 29g; Fiber: 5g; Protein: 41g; Calcium: 381mg; Sodium: 812mg; Potassium: 865mg; Vitamin D: 1mcg; Iron: 5mg; Zinc: 7mg

# Marinated Grilled Pepper Flank Steak

✔ BUDGET-SAVER

✔ ONE-POT

**SERVES 2**

**PREP TIME:** 15 MINUTES,
PLUS 1 HOUR TO MARINATE

**COOK TIME:** 15 MINUTES

½ teaspoon garlic powder

¼ teaspoon ground cumin

¼ teaspoon freshly ground black pepper

10 ounces beef flank steak

2 tablespoons balsamic vinegar

2 tablespoons reduced-sodium soy sauce

2 teaspoons honey

1 teaspoon avocado oil

¼ teaspoon cayenne pepper (optional)

Flank steak is an inexpensive cut of beef, and when cooked properly, it is delicious. The prep is quick, but you'll want to allow at least an hour for marinating, which seals in the juices. Using a reduced-sodium soy sauce adds flavor without adding much salt. Try serving this tender steak with a green salad or with the Bold Bean Shrimp Fiesta Salad (page 45).

1. In a small bowl, combine the garlic powder, cumin, and pepper. Rub the spice blend all over the steak and set aside.

2. Combine the vinegar, soy sauce, honey, oil, and cayenne pepper (if using) in a large zip-top plastic bag.

3. Add the flank steak to the bag, squeeze out the excess air, and seal. Marinate the steak in the refrigerator for an hour (or for up to 12 hours, turning it over occasionally and moving the marinade around it to ensure that it's marinating evenly).

4. Preheat a grill to medium-high heat for 10 minutes. Remove the marinated steak from the bag. Discard the marinade and place the steak on the grill. Grill for 3 minutes per side for medium-rare or 4 minutes per side for medium.

5. If you do not have a grill, sear the steak on a griddle or in a skillet over high heat for 3 minutes per side.

6. Allow the steak to rest for 5 to 10 minutes. Cut it against the grain into ¼-inch-thick slices and serve.

CONTINUED ▶

## Marinated Grilled Pepper Flank Steak CONTINUED

**PREP TIP:** Cook times vary depending on the thickness of the steak. You can check doneness using a meat thermometer. For medium-rare, the internal temperature is 120°F to 125°F, and for medium, it's 130°F to 135°F.

**STORAGE TIP:** Store in an airtight container in the refrigerator for up to 3 days.

. . . . . . . . . . . . . . . . . . . . . . . . . . . . . . . . . . . . . . . . . . . . . . . . . . . .

**Per Serving**  Calories: 261; Total fat: 9g; Carbohydrates: 10g; Fiber: 0g; Protein: 32g; Calcium: 42mg; Sodium: 591mg; Potassium: 569mg; Vitamin D: 0mcg; Iron: 3mg; Zinc: 6mg

# 50-50 Burgers with Caramelized Onions

✔ **30 MINUTES OR LESS**
✔ **BUDGET-SAVER**
✔ **ONE-POT**

**SERVES 2**

**PREP TIME:** 10 MINUTES
**COOK TIME:** 20 MINUTES

1 cup finely chopped white mushrooms

¼ teaspoon olive oil

¾ cup sliced onions

4 ounces 90 percent lean ground beef

1 teaspoon Steak and Chop salt-free seasoning blend

⅛ teaspoon salt

2 hard rolls

Have you heard of "The Blend"? It's a method using part mushrooms and part meat to make burgers, tacos, or chilis. This reduces your overall meal cost, adds a healthy vegetable to your diet, and reduces the fat in the burger. The mushrooms blend in so well with the beef you'll hardly notice them at all. I like to sauté the mushrooms first to make the burgers nice and juicy.

1. Heat a large nonstick skillet over medium heat. Add the mushrooms and cook for about 3 minutes or until soft. Drain off any water, transfer the mushrooms to a large bowl, and set them aside.

2. Heat the oil in the same skillet over medium heat, add the onions, and sauté until translucent, about 3 minutes. Reduce the heat to low and cook until the onions are caramelized, about 15 minutes.

3. While the onions cook, add the beef, seasoning, and salt to the mushrooms. Mix thoroughly and divide the mixture into two burgers.

4. Transfer the caramelized onions to a small bowl and set aside.

5. Increase the heat to medium-high and put the same skillet back on the heat. Place the burgers in the skillet and cook them for 7 to 10 minutes, turning once.

6. Serve the burgers topped with the onions on the hard rolls. Feel free to add other vegetable toppings, such as sliced tomato, leaf lettuce, or spinach.

CONTINUED ▶

**SUBSTITUTION TIP:** You can substitute ground turkey for the beef.

**PREP TIP:** You can also cook these burgers on a preheated grill for 4 minutes per side.

. . . . . . . . . . . . . . . . . . . . . . . . . . . . . . . . . . . . . . . . . . . . . . . . . .

**Per Serving** Calories: 297; Total fat: 9g; Carbohydrates: 35g; Fiber: 2g; Protein: 19g; Calcium: 72mg; Sodium: 506mg; Potassium: 418mg; Vitamin D: 0mcg; Iron: 3mg; Zinc: 4mg

# Beef Fajitas

✔ **30 MINUTES OR LESS**
✔ **BUDGET-SAVER**
✔ **ONE-POT**

**SERVES 2**

**PREP TIME:** 10 MINUTES
**COOK TIME:** 15 MINUTES

1 teaspoon canola oil

6 ounces beef sirloin, sliced thinly

2 teaspoons salt-free Tex-Mex seasoning

2 bell peppers, sliced

½ medium onion, sliced

4 (6-inch) flour tortillas

1 avocado, peeled, pitted, and sliced

¼ cup shredded sharp cheddar cheese

½ cup nonfat Greek yogurt

1 lime, cut into 4 wedges

This take on classic fajitas uses a smaller portion of lean beef that's cooked up with a load of peppers and onions, making it DASH-friendly. Reduce the sodium even further by using corn tortillas in place of the flour ones. If you're looking to reduce calories, use Bibb lettuce leaves in place of the tortillas. Avocado adds a festive feel to the dish as well as healthy monounsaturated fat.

1.  Heat the oil in a large nonstick skillet over medium heat. Add the sliced beef, sprinkle it with the seasoning, and stir to distribute. Sauté the beef for 3 minutes, stirring to brown both sides. Add the peppers and onions, cover, and let cook for 2 minutes. Stir, replace the lid, and cook until the vegetables are tender.

2.  Wrap the tortillas in a paper towel and heat them in the microwave for 30 seconds. Or, you can wrap them in foil and heat them in a 170°F oven for 3 to 5 minutes.

3.  Divide the beef between the 4 tortillas. Top each with avocado, cheese, and the peppers and onions. Garnish with a dollop of yogurt and a lime wedge and serve.

**SUBSTITUTION TIP:** If you can't find salt-free Tex-Mex seasoning, use: ½ teaspoon cumin, 1 teaspoon chili powder, and ¼ teaspoon cayenne pepper. You can also substitute ¼ cup of light sour cream for the ½ cup of yogurt.

**VARIATION TIP:** You can substitute chicken for the beef.

**STORAGE TIP:** Store in an airtight container in the refrigerator for up to 3 days.

. . . . . . . . . . . . . . . . . . . . . . . . . . . . . . . . . . . . . . . . . . . . . . .

**Per Serving** Calories: 691; Total fat: 36g; Carbohydrates: 59g; Fiber: 12g; Protein: 37g; Calcium: 296mg; Sodium: 590mg; Potassium: 1219mg; Vitamin D: 0mcg; Iron: 4mg; Zinc: 5mg

# Vegged-Up Beef Enchilada Casserole

✔ BUDGET-SAVER
✔ ONE-POT

**SERVES 3 TO 4**

**PREP TIME:** 15 MINUTES
**COOK TIME:** 20 MINUTES

Nonstick cooking spray

1 (15-ounce) can pure pumpkin purée

½ cup low-sodium beef broth

4 tablespoons tomato paste, divided

1½ teaspoons chili powder, divided

¾ teaspoon cumin, divided

¼ teaspoon cayenne pepper (optional)

½ teaspoon olive oil

8 ounces extra lean ground beef

1 cup canned pinto beans, drained and rinsed

½ cup water

4 (8-inch) flour tortillas

⅓ cup shredded sharp cheddar cheese

½ cup nonfat Greek yogurt, for garnish

These "pumped" up enchiladas get extra nutrition by using pumpkin purée in the creamy, bright-hued sauce. Pumpkin is loaded with beta carotene and other antioxidants as well as fiber. Store-bought enchilada sauces, both tomato- and cream-based, are extremely high in sodium. Making your own sauce with a unique twist means you can enjoy this fabulous dish regularly.

1. Preheat the oven to 350°F. Spray an 8-by-8-inch baking dish with cooking spray.

2. In a small saucepan, stir together the pumpkin, broth, 2 tablespoons tomato paste, 1 teaspoon chili powder, ½ teaspoon cumin, and the cayenne pepper (if using) until well blended. Heat the sauce over medium-high heat until it begins to boil, then remove it from the heat and set it aside. If the sauce seems to be too thick, stir in a little water.

3. In a large skillet, heat the oil over medium-high heat. Brown the beef for 7 to 8 minutes, then drain off any fat. Add the beans, water, and the remaining tomato paste, chili powder, and cumin and stir. Cook until heated through.

4. Spread ½ cup of the sauce over the bottom of the prepared baking dish. On a clean surface or cutting board, lay a tortilla flat, add ¼ of the beef mixture, then roll tightly and place in the bottom of the prepared dish. Do the same with the other 3 tortillas.

5. Pour the remaining sauce over the filled tortillas, covering them evenly. Sprinkle the shredded cheese over the sauce.

6. Bake for 20 to 25 minutes and serve garnished with dollops of yogurt.

**SUBSTITUTION TIP:** You can use ground pork, turkey, or chicken in place of the beef. Or you can omit the meat and just use 3 cups of pinto beans.

**STORAGE TIP:** Store in an airtight container in the refrigerator for up to 3 days.

. . . . . . . . . . . . . . . . . . . . . . . . . . . . . . . . . . . . . . . . . . . . . . . . . . .

**Per Serving** Calories: 566; Total fat: 18g; Carbohydrates: 66g; Fiber: 12g; Protein: 36g; Calcium: 316mg; Sodium: 681mg; Potassium: 1019mg; Vitamin D: 0mcg; Iron: 8mg; Zinc: 6mg

# Rigatoni with Bolognese Sauce

✔ BUDGET-SAVER

✔ MAKE-AHEAD

✔ ONE-POT

**SERVES 2 TO 3**

**PREP TIME:** 20 MINUTES

**COOK TIME:** 1 HOUR,
10 MINUTES

6 ounces 90 percent lean
  ground beef

1 garlic clove, pressed
  or minced

½ teaspoon olive oil

¾ cup finely
  chopped carrots

¼ cup diced onion

½ cup white wine

1½ cups water

1 (6-ounce) can
  tomato paste

1 teaspoon chopped
  fresh parsley or
  ½ teaspoon dried

6 ounces rigatoni

Freshly ground
  black pepper

2 tablespoons grated
  Parmesan cheese,
  for garnish

This classic pasta dish meets DASH diet guidelines because the portion of beef per serving is small. The lycopene-rich tomatoes add antioxidants as well as potassium. I also snuck a few extra carrots in for added nutrition. You'll want to use a sturdy pasta like rigatoni or penne for this sauce, as wimpy slender noodles will not hold up. Simmering the sauce longer deepens the favor, so allow extra time when making this delicious meal.

1. Heat a large saucepan over medium-high heat. Add the beef and cook, stirring to break up larger pieces, until it is browned and no pink remains. Add the garlic and cook for 1 more minute. Remove the beef from the saucepan and set it aside in a small bowl.

2. Heat the oil in the same saucepan over medium heat. Add the carrots and onion and sauté for 2 to 3 minutes.

3. Add the beef back to the saucepan, then add the wine. Simmer until the wine evaporates, 3 to 4 minutes.

4. Reduce the heat to low and add the water, tomato paste, and parsley, stirring until combined. Cover and allow the sauce to simmer on very low heat for at least 1 hour or up to 3 hours.

5. When you're ready to eat, fill a large stockpot three-quarters full with water and bring it to a boil over high heat. Cook the pasta in the boiling water as directed on the package.

6. Drain the pasta (don't rinse it), and then add it to the sauce.

7. Season with pepper to taste and serve garnished with the Parmesan cheese.

**SUBSTITUTION TIP:** Tagliatelle or fettuccine pasta works well with this sauce, too.

**STORAGE TIP:** Store in an airtight container in the refrigerator for up to 3 days.

. . . . . . . . . . . . . . . . . . . . . . . . . . . . . . . . . . . . . . . . . . . . . . . . . . .

**Per Serving** Calories: 646; Total fat: 13g; Carbohydrates: 88g; Fiber: 8g; Protein: 34g; Calcium: 113mg; Sodium: 239mg; Potassium: 1468mg; Vitamin D: 0mcg; Iron: 6mg; Zinc: 6mg

# Slow-Cooker Beef Round with Vegetables

✔ MAKE-AHEAD
✔ ONE-POT

**SERVES 2 TO 3**

**PREP TIME:** 15 MINUTES
**COOK TIME:** 3 HOURS

10 ounces beef round steak, cut into bite-size pieces

3 tablespoons all-purpose flour

1 cup low-sodium beef broth

¼ cup balsamic vinegar

2 tablespoons tomato paste

¾ pound medley small potatoes (red, yellow, purple)

1½ cups roughly chopped carrots

½ onion, sliced

½ cup chopped, sun-dried tomatoes

½ cup water

2 teaspoons dried rosemary

½ teaspoon garlic powder

Coming home to a favorite slow-cooked meal is always gratifying. This rich beef stew gets its robust taste from sun-dried tomatoes. You can add any potato to it, but I used a medley of small yellow, purple, and red mini potatoes. Some slow-cooker recipes call for browning the beef before adding it to the slow cooker, but for a stew, you can save time by skipping that step.

1. In a medium bowl, toss the beef cubes with the flour to lightly coat.

2. In a small bowl, combine the broth, vinegar, and tomato paste until well mixed.

3. Put the potatoes, carrots, onion, beef, sun-dried tomatoes, water, rosemary, garlic powder, and broth mixture in the slow cooker.

4. Cover and cook on high for 3 hours or on low for 6 hours.

**INGREDIENT TIP:** Roasts are usually about 3 pounds. You can always cut a large roast in half and freeze one portion for up to 3 months. Your grocer may also sell round steak in smaller packages and already cut into stew cubes.

**STORAGE TIP:** Store in an airtight container in the refrigerator for up to 3 days.

. . . . . . . . . . . . . . . . . . . . . . . . . . . . . . . . . . . . . . . . . . . .

**Per Serving** Calories: 474; Total fat: 7g; Carbohydrates: 64g; Fiber: 9g; Protein: 40g; Calcium: 94mg; Sodium: 237mg; Potassium: 2012mg; Vitamin D: 0mcg; Iron: 8mg; Zinc: 7mg

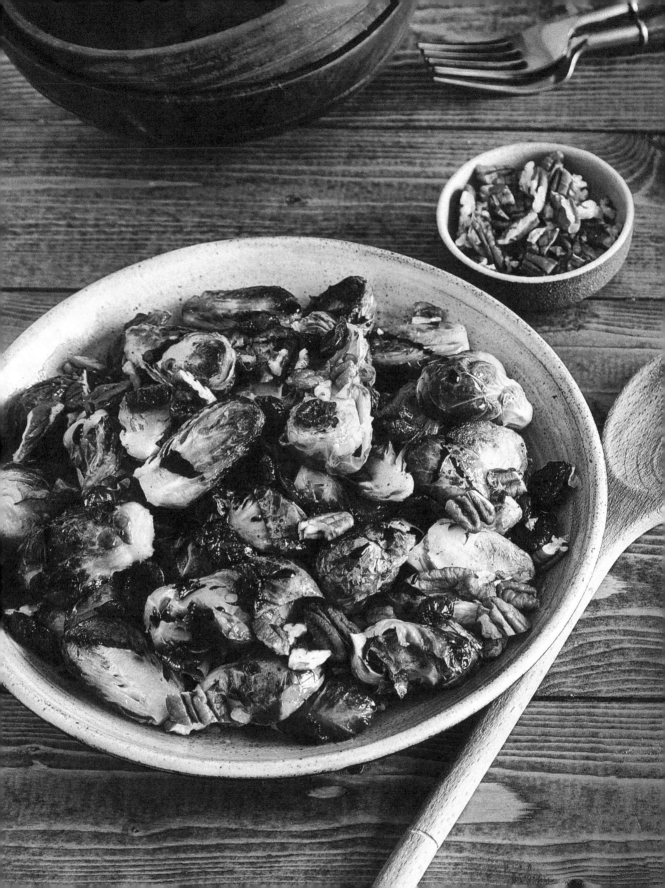

# 9
# SIDES

# Beans and Greens

✔ 30 MINUTES OR LESS
✔ BUDGET-SAVER
✔ ONE-POT
✔ VEGETARIAN

**SERVES 2 TO 3**

**PREP TIME:** 10 MINUTES
**COOK TIME:** 15 MINUTES

2 teaspoons olive oil

2 garlic cloves, pressed
or minced

1 large bunch escarole

Pinch salt

¼ teaspoon red
pepper flakes

1 (15-ounce) can cannelloni
beans, drained and rinsed

1 tablespoon grated
Parmesan
cheese (optional)

If you are from the Southern United States, this dish might stir some memories, as braised collard greens and pinto beans are a signature dish in that region. Escarole takes the place of the heartier green in this healthy Italian-inspired side dish, and you won't see the ubiquitous piece of fatback simmering in your pot. This version offers potassium, folate, and other B vitamins, as well as iron, fiber, and protein. It's delicious alongside fish or roast chicken and is satisfying enough to be a main dish served with barley or rice.

1. Heat the oil in a large skillet over medium heat. Add the garlic and sauté for 1 to 2 minutes; do not brown it. Reduce the heat to low, and add the greens, salt, and red pepper flakes. Stir and then cover and cook for 4 minutes, or until the greens are wilted.

2. Add the beans and stir to combine. Cook for 7 to 10 minutes, stirring occasionally.

3. Garnish with the Parmesan (if using) and serve.

**INGREDIENT TIP:** Don't rinse the beans for this recipe. The starch helps the ingredients come together to provide a light "sauce."

. . . . . . . . . . . . . . . . . . . . . . . . . . . . . . . . . . . . . . . . . . . . . .

**Per Serving** Calories: 225; Total fat: 5g; Carbohydrates: 34g; Fiber: 15g; Protein: 13g; Calcium: 145mg; Sodium: 104mg; Potassium: 843mg; Vitamin D: 0mcg; Iron: 5mg; Zinc: 2mg

# Garlicky Roasted Broccoli

✓ **ONE-POT**

✓ **VEGAN**

**SERVES 2 TO 3**

**PREP TIME:** 10 MINUTES

**COOK TIME:** 30 MINUTES

1 bunch broccoli, cut into small florets

3 garlic cloves, pressed or minced

2 teaspoons olive oil

Pinch salt

Many people complain that vegetables don't have enough flavor. But roasting vegetables such as broccoli brings out their natural sugars. Layering ingredients also helps boost flavor (along with lots of garlic!) and retain texture. Broccoli provides you with a good dose of potassium, folate, vitamin C, beta carotene, and other antioxidants.

1. Preheat the oven to 400°F. Line a baking sheet with parchment paper.

2. Spread the broccoli and garlic onto the baking sheet.

3. Drizzle the vegetables with olive oil, sprinkle them with salt, and toss together.

4. Bake for 30 minutes until tender, stirring midway through the cooking time, and serve.

**PREP TIP:** To make florets, cut the large stem from the broccoli, then gently break off florets with your fingers. Use a knife to cut the stalks from larger florets. You can also slice the stalk into thin slices and roast those as well.

**STORAGE TIP:** Store in an airtight container in the refrigerator for up to 3 days.

. . . . . . . . . . . . . . . . . . . . . . . . . . . . . . . . . . . . . . . . . . . . . . . . . . . .

**Per Serving** Calories: 150; Total fat: 6g; Carbohydrates: 22g; Fiber: 8g; Protein: 9g; Calcium: 151mg; Sodium: 179mg; Potassium: 879mg; Vitamin D: 0mcg; Iron: 2mg; Zinc: 1mg

# Sautéed Zucchini with Onions

✔ 30 MINUTES OR LESS
✔ BUDGET-SAVER
✔ ONE-POT
✔ VEGAN

**SERVES 2 TO 3**

**PREP TIME:** 5 MINUTES
**COOK TIME:** 10 MINUTES

½ teaspoon olive oil

2 small zucchini, sliced

½ onion, thinly sliced

Pinch salt

Pinch freshly ground
  black pepper

Zucchini cooks up quickly in this simple side dish. The unique texture and fresh summery flavor of the vegetable are not hidden in a sauce or overpowered by other ingredients. Zucchini is low-calorie but is high in A, C, and B vitamins as well as magnesium and potassium. This speedy side pairs well with just about any entrée. Try it with Lemon Caper Pork Cutlets (page 145) or the Pork Tenderloin Medallions with Dijon–Yogurt Sauce (page 142).

1. Heat the oil over medium heat in a large nonstick skillet.

2. Add the zucchini and onions to the skillet. Cover and let cook for 3 minutes.

3. Uncover, stir, and add the salt and pepper. Continuing cooking until tender, for about 2 to 3 more minutes, and serve.

**VARIATION TIP:** Add ½ teaspoon of red pepper flakes if you enjoy it hot, or, if you don't, add ½ teaspoon of Herbs de Provence.

. . . . . . . . . . . . . . . . . . . . . . . . . . . . . . . . . . . . . . . . . . .

**Per Serving** Calories: 59; Total fat: 2g; Carbohydrates: 10g; Fiber: 3g; Protein: 3g; Calcium: 41mg; Sodium: 95mg; Potassium: 570mg; Vitamin D: 0mcg; Iron: 1mg; Zinc: 1mg

# Roasted Brussels Sprouts with Dried Cranberries

✔ **BUDGET-SAVER**
✔ **ONE-POT**
✔ **VEGAN**

**SERVES 2 TO 3**

**PREP TIME:** 15 MINUTES
**COOK TIME:** 35 MINUTES

Nonstick cooking spray

3 cups halved
 Brussels sprouts

Pinch salt

2 teaspoons olive oil

¼ cup dried cranberries

½ cup chopped pecans

2 teaspoons balsamic glaze

Roasting veggies takes a little time in the oven, but it mellows and enhances their natural flavor, since they can be slightly bitter otherwise. This cruciferous veggie isn't just heart-healthy—it's also linked to reducing the risk of colon cancer. The cranberries and nuts add some additional sweetness and texture to the dish.

1. Preheat the oven to 400°F. Spray a baking sheet with cooking spray.

2. Place the Brussels sprouts on the baking sheet, drizzle with olive oil, and sprinkle with salt.

3. Roast the veggies for 20 minutes. Toss the sprouts and add the cranberries and nuts. Continue roasting for an additional 15 minutes until the sprouts are lightly browned. Transfer them to a serving bowl.

4. Drizzle the Brussels sprouts with the balsamic glaze and serve.

**STORAGE TIP:** Store in an airtight container in the refrigerator for up to 3 days.

. . . . . . . . . . . . . . . . . . . . . . . . . . . . . . . . . . . . . . . . . . . . . . . .

**Per Serving** Calories: 337; Total fat: 24g; Carbohydrates: 29g; Fiber: 9g; Protein: 7g; Calcium: 78mg; Sodium: 112mg; Potassium: 637mg; Vitamin D: 0mcg; Iron: 3mg; Zinc: 2mg

# Roasted Asparagus with Lemon

✔ **30 MINUTES OR LESS**

✔ **ONE-POT**

✔ **VEGAN**

**SERVES 2**

**PREP TIME:** 10 MINUTES
**COOK TIME:** 20 MINUTES

1 bunch asparagus,
  ends trimmed

1 teaspoon olive oil

Pinch salt

1 lemon

Asparagus is another vegetable that lends itself to roasting. It's also great grilled. Pop these into the oven to roast, then add a flavor-brightening squeeze of lemon, and you have a healthy and delicious side dish. This is a good side to serve with the Lemon Caper Pork Cutlets (page 145) or the Quick Chicken Marsala (page 122) because the flavors are complementary.

1. Preheat the oven to 400°F. Line a baking sheet with parchment paper.

2. Spread the asparagus on the baking sheet; drizzle it with oil and sprinkle it with salt. Grate some lemon zest over the asparagus, about ¼ of the lemon.

3. Roast the asparagus for 20 minutes, tossing halfway through.

4. Squeeze some lemon juice onto the cooked asparagus before serving.

5. Garnish with lemon slices if desired.

**PREP TIP:** To remove the woody ends of the asparagus, simply bend the stalk. The stalk will snap right where it gets tough and stringy.

. . . . . . . . . . . . . . . . . . . . . . . . . . . . . . . . . . . . . . . . . . . . . . . . . .

**Per Serving** Calories: 44; Total fat: 2g; Carbohydrates: 5g; Fiber: 2g; Protein: 2g; Calcium: 25mg; Sodium: 80mg; Potassium: 218mg; Vitamin D: 0mcg; Iron: 2mg; Zinc: 1mg

# Herbed Air-Fried Zucchini Planks

✔ **30 MINUTES OR LESS**

✔ **ONE-POT**

✔ **VEGETARIAN**

**SERVES 2 TO 3**

**PREP TIME:** 15 MINUTES

**COOK TIME:** 10 MINUTES

¼ cup all-purpose flour

1 large egg

¼ cup 1 percent milk

1 cup bread crumbs

1 teaspoon Herbs
de Provence

½ teaspoon dried oregano

Pinch salt

Pinch freshly ground
black pepper

2 small zucchini, sliced
lengthwise into
¼-inch planks

Nonstick cooking spray

Air fryers are common in many kitchens these days. Using this device ensures that these zucchini planks have fewer calories because you use less oil than in the traditional fried version. Plus, they take almost no time to air-fry. If you don't have an air fryer, no problem. (See tip.)

1. Preheat an oven-style air fryer to 400°F.

2. Put the flour in a shallow plate or bowl.

3. In a small bowl, whisk the egg and milk together.

4. In another small bowl, stir together the bread crumbs, Herbs de Provence, oregano, salt, and pepper.

5. Dip the zucchini planks, one at a time, into the flour, then the egg mixture, then into the bread crumbs, lightly covering both sides. Transfer the planks to the air-fryer tray as you bread them.

6. Spray the zucchini evenly with cooking spray. Air-fry the planks for 8 to 10 minutes, turning them over halfway through the cooking time. Serve immediately.

**COOKING TIP:** If you don't have an air fryer, preheat the oven to 425°F. Place the planks on a baking sheet sprayed with oil and bake them for 25 to 30 minutes, turning them halfway through the cooking time.

. . . . . . . . . . . . . . . . . . . . . . . . . . . . . . . . . . . . . . . . . . . . . . . . . . . .

**Per Serving** Calories: 376; Total fat: 7g; Carbohydrates: 63g; Fiber: 6g; Protein: 16g; Calcium: 209mg; Sodium: 512mg; Potassium: 1049mg; Vitamin D: 1mcg; Iron: 5mg; Zinc: 2mg

# Cauliflower Mash with Garlic-Yogurt Cream

✔ **30 MINUTES OR LESS**
✔ **MAKE-AHEAD**
✔ **VEGETARIAN**

**SERVES 2 TO 3**

**PREP TIME:** 10 MINUTES
**COOK TIME:** 15 MINUTES

3 cups water

½ teaspoon olive oil

1 head of cauliflower, stem removed and grated or finely chopped

2 garlic cloves, pressed or minced

¾ cup nonfat Greek yogurt

There is nothing wrong with a good mashed potato, but mashed cauliflower can add a little variety to your diet. If you have never tried mashed cauliflower in place of mashed potatoes, the similarly fluffy texture of whipped cauliflower might surprise you. An immersion blender gives this dish a creamier texture, but you can use a potato masher instead if you don't have the tool. You can make this ahead, store it in an oven-safe dish, and then reheat it in a 300°F oven for 15 minutes.

*1.* Bring the water to a boil in a large stockpot over high heat.

*2.* While the water boils, heat the olive oil in a large skillet over medium-high heat. Add the cauliflower and garlic. Sauté for 3 to 4 minutes.

*3.* Transfer the cauliflower and garlic to the boiling water and boil for 10 minutes.

*4.* Drain the cauliflower and return it to the stockpot. Add the yogurt and blend until smooth with an immersion blender or food processor, then serve.

**PREP TIP:** When boiling the cauliflower, only use enough water to just cover it, so the dish doesn't end up too mushy.

**STORAGE TIP:** Store in an airtight container in the refrigerator for up to 3 days.

. . . . . . . . . . . . . . . . . . . . . . . . . . . . . . . . . . . . . . . . . . . . . . .

**Per Serving** Calories: 138; Total fat: 2g; Carbohydrates: 19g; Fiber: 6g; Protein: 15g; Calcium: 164mg; Sodium: 119mg; Potassium: 911mg; Vitamin D: 0mcg; Iron: 1mg; Zinc: 1mg

# Brown Rice with Herbs de Provence

✓ ONE-POT

**SERVES 2**

**PREP TIME:** 10 MINUTES
**COOK TIME:** 50 MINUTES

½ cup brown rice

½ teaspoon olive oil

1 cup low-sodium
   chicken broth

1 teaspoon Herbs
   de Provence

Brown rice has a mildly nutty flavor and more fiber than white rice. Fiber helps you stay full and lowers your blood lipids. By skipping the boxed rice mixes, you'll save sodium but not skimp on flavor. This dish is flavored with olive oil and herbs, and cooking the rice in chicken stock adds a rich taste, as well. You can switch out the herbs for other favorites, but the Herbs de Provence blend gives an aromatic, slightly floral character to the dish.

1. Put the rice into a mesh colander and rinse it under cold water.

2. Heat the oil in a large saucepan over medium heat. Add the rice and stir quickly to toast it for 1 to 2 minutes. Add the broth and Herbs de Provence and bring the mixture to a boil. Reduce the heat to low, cover, and simmer for 40 to 45 minutes, until all liquid is absorbed. Remove the rice from the heat and keep it covered for 10 more minutes.

3. Fluff the rice gently with a fork and serve.

**SUBSTITUTION TIP:** To save time, you can use instant brown rice and follow the package directions. To make this vegan, use vegetable broth.

**STORAGE TIP:** Store in an airtight container in the refrigerator for up to 3 days.

. . . . . . . . . . . . . . . . . . . . . . . . . . . . . . . . . . . . . . . . . . . . . . . . . . . .

**Per Serving** Calories: 182; Total fat: 2g; Carbohydrates: 36g; Fiber: 2g; Protein: 4g; Calcium: 16mg; Sodium: 2mg; Potassium: 127mg; Vitamin D: 0mcg; Iron: 1mg; Zinc: 1mg

# Curried Vegetable Rice

✓ 30 MINUTES OR LESS
✓ VEGAN

**SERVES 2 TO 3**

**PREP TIME:** 5 MINUTES
**COOK TIME:** 15 MINUTES

½ cup instant brown rice

1 teaspoon curry powder

1 cup chopped carrots

1 cup green beans, cut into 1-inch pieces

1 teaspoon olive oil

¼ cup chopped onions

¼ teaspoon garlic powder

Side dishes don't have to be fancy or use numerous ingredients to be fabulous. Adding a few basic veggies to rice amplifies its nutrition profile and creates a more flavorful dish. Of course, the piquant curry powder ensures that this side will hold its own with any entrée. Using instant rice gets this dish onto the table quickly, so you can enjoy it at any time.

1. Cook the rice according to the package directions with the addition of the curry powder, about 5 minutes.

2. While the rice cooks, put the carrots and green beans into a large skillet. Add ½ cup of water, place the skillet over medium-high heat, cover it, and steam the vegetables for 5 minutes until they are tender-crisp.

3. Drain the water from the skillet, add the oil, onions, and garlic powder, and cook for 3 more minutes.

4. Add the vegetables to the cooked rice. Fluff with a fork and serve.

**SUBSTITUTION TIP:** You can use a variety of cooked vegetables for this dish, including zucchini, broccoli, bell peppers, or mushrooms.

**STORAGE TIP:** Store in an airtight container in the refrigerator for up to 3 days.

. . . . . . . . . . . . . . . . . . . . . . . . . . . . . . . . . . . . . . . . . . . . . . . . . . . .

**Per Serving** Calories: 246; Total fat: 4g; Carbohydrates: 49g; Fiber: 6g; Protein: 6g; Calcium: 65mg; Sodium: 51mg; Potassium: 483mg; Vitamin D: 0mcg; Iron: 2mg; Zinc: 1mg

# DASH Twice-Baked Potatoes

✓ **MAKE-AHEAD**

✓ **ONE-POT**

**SERVES 2 TO 3**

**PREP TIME:** 15 MINUTES

**COOK TIME:** 55 MINUTES

2 large potatoes

1 teaspoon avocado oil

½ cup nonfat Greek yogurt

¼ teaspoon white
  ground pepper

Pinch salt

½ teaspoon paprika

3 tablespoons shredded
  sharp cheddar cheese

Did you know that a potato has more potassium than a banana and almost as much vitamin C as an orange? Because of this, potatoes are definitely DASH-friendly. This lightened-up version of twice-baked spuds also incorporates yogurt to help you meet your dairy servings. Serve these flavor-packed potatoes alongside Bass with Citrus Butter (page 108) or the Pork Tenderloin Medallions with Dijon–Yogurt Sauce (page 142).

1. Preheat the oven to 400°F.

2. Bake the potatoes directly on the oven rack for 40 minutes. Remove the potatoes from the oven and let them cool until you can handle them.

3. Cut each potato in half. Scoop out the potato flesh, up to about ¼-inch from the skin, and transfer the flesh to a small bowl. Add the oil and mash. Set the empty skins aside.

4. Mix the yogurt, pepper, and salt into the potato flesh and whip it with a spoon. Once it's well-combined, spoon the mixture back into the potato skins. Top with a sprinkling of paprika. Divide the cheese evenly between the filled potatoes.

5. Place the potatoes on a baking sheet and bake for another 15 minutes, until lightly browned on top, and serve.

**PREP TIP:** You can double the recipe and freeze these after step 4. The frozen potatoes can be baked in a 350°F oven for 25 minutes to reheat.

. . . . . . . . . . . . . . . . . . . . . . . . . . . . . . . . . . . . . . . . . . . . . .

**Per Serving** Calories: 385; Total fat: 7g; Carbohydrates: 67g; Fiber: 8g; Protein: 16g; Calcium: 184mg; Sodium: 193mg; Potassium: 1324mg; Vitamin D: 0mcg; Iron: 3mg; Zinc: 2mg

# Sweet Potato Steak Fries

✔ **30 MINUTES OR LESS**
✔ **ONE-POT**
✔ **VEGAN**

**SERVES 2 TO 3**

**PREP TIME:** 10 MINUTES
**COOK TIME:** 20 MINUTES

2 sweet potatoes, peeled and cut lengthwise into ¼-inch batons

¼ teaspoon cornstarch

1 teaspoon avocado oil

½ teaspoon salt-free mesquite seasoning

⅛ teaspoon salt

Sweet potato fries are a trendy dish that's served everywhere, from food carts to Michelin-star restaurants, for a good reason. The natural sweetness of this ingredient is concentrated when the vegetable caramelizes in the heat. When combined with seasonings, the flavor explodes in your mouth. Sweet potatoes are an excellent source of disease-fighting beta carotene, which is an added benefit.

1. Heat the oven to 425°F. Line a baking sheet with parchment paper or a silicone mat.

2. Put the potatoes in a small mixing bowl and sprinkle them with the cornstarch, coating the batons evenly. Drizzle the avocado oil into the bowl and toss the potatoes to coat. Add the seasoning and salt and toss to combine.

3. Transfer the potatoes to the baking sheet and bake for 15 to 20 minutes, turning after 10 minutes. Serve hot.

**PREP TIP:** For a crispier potato, air-fry the sweet potatoes for 8 minutes at 425°F.

. . . . . . . . . . . . . . . . . . . . . . . . . . . . . . . . . . . . . . . . . . . . . . . .

**Per Serving** Calories: 133; Total fat: 2g; Carbohydrates: 26g; Fiber: 4g; Protein: 2g; Calcium: 39mg; Sodium: 227mg; Potassium: 438mg; Vitamin D: 0mcg; Iron: 1mg; Zinc: 0mg

# Roasted Potato Party

✔ ONE-POT
✔ VEGAN

**SERVES 2 TO 3**

**PREP TIME:** 5 MINUTES
**COOK TIME:** 45 MINUTES

1 (24-ounce) bag medley potatoes, scrubbed

2 teaspoons olive oil

1 teaspoon dried rosemary

½ teaspoon garlic powder

Pinch salt

1 tablespoon chopped parsley, for garnish (optional)

The color variety of these medley potatoes makes them party-worthy, but their nutritional profile makes them DASH-friendly. All potatoes are potassium-rich, but the different colors in medley potatoes signify different nutrients; the deep purple potatoes are full of anthocyanins (an antioxidant giving them their color), and the yellow ones are higher in beta carotene. These antioxidants are good for both your heart and brain. Feel free to invite the Sheet Pan Chicken Thighs (page 119) over.

1. Preheat the oven to 400°F. Line a baking sheet with parchment paper.

2. In a medium bowl, toss the potatoes with the oil, rosemary, garlic powder, and salt.

3. Spread the potatoes on the baking sheet and bake for 35 to 45 minutes, tossing halfway through the cooking time.

4. Sprinkle the roasted potatoes with the parsley (if using) and serve.

**VARIATION TIP:** Make this party even more fun by adding cubed parsnips and carrots.

**STORAGE TIP:** Store in an airtight container in the refrigerator for up to 3 days.

. . . . . . . . . . . . . . . . . . . . . . . . . . . . . . . . . . . . . . . . . . . . . . . . . . . . . . . .

**Per Serving** Calories: 306; Total fat: 5g; Carbohydrates: 60g; Fiber: 8g; Protein: 7g; Calcium: 49mg; Sodium: 99mg; Potassium: 1148mg; Vitamin D: 0mcg; Iron: 3mg; Zinc: 1mg

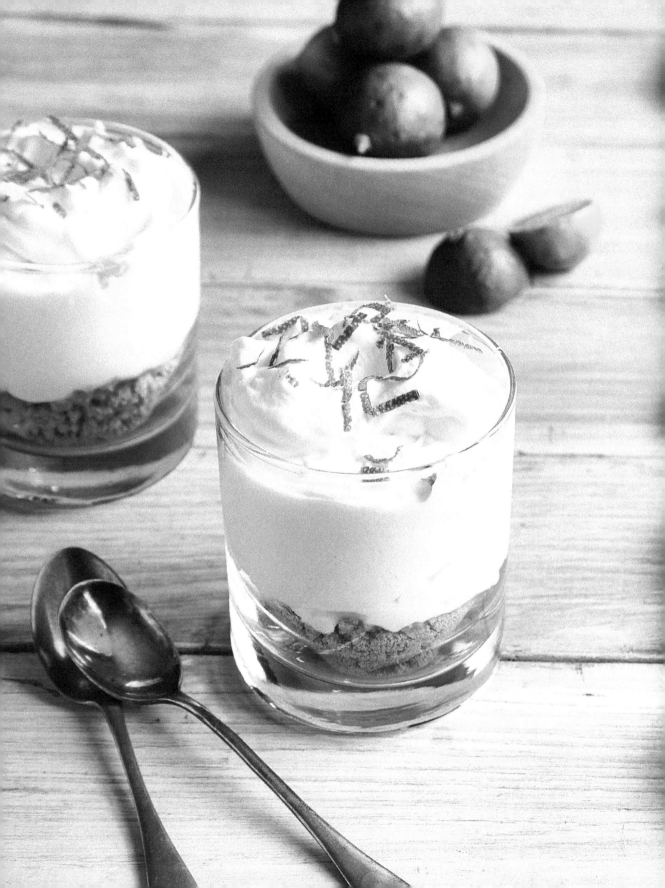

# 10
# DESSERTS AND SWEETS

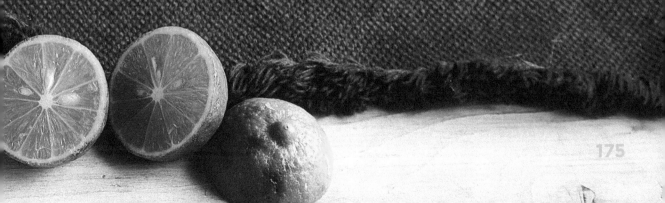

# Greek Yogurt Key Lime Cups

✔ ONE-POT

✔ VEGETARIAN

**SERVES 2**

**PREP TIME:** 20 MINUTES

1 graham cracker sheet

2 ounces light cream cheese, softened

½ cup nonfat Greek yogurt

2½ tablespoons key lime juice, bottled or fresh

2 teaspoons honey

Canned whipped cream, for garnish

1 teaspoon grated lime zest, for garnish (optional)

Desserts aren't a focus of DASH, but you can certainly enjoy a sweet treat now and then. This recipe creates a sweet cheesecake-like creation flavored with tart lime juice and honey. Even better, you can eat it guilt-free regularly. This fluffy dessert doesn't require baking, so it is easy to make. It does require some refrigeration time, so plan on making it ahead.

1. Place the graham cracker between two pieces of wax paper, then crush it with a rolling pin. Divide the crumbs between two dessert cups.

2. In a medium bowl, beat the cream cheese, yogurt, lime juice, and honey with an electric hand mixer or whisk until smooth.

3. Spoon the mixture into the dessert cups and refrigerate for an hour.

4. When ready to serve, garnish with whipped cream and lime zest (if using).

**SUBSTITUTION TIP:** Try key lime flavored Greek yogurt in place of the plain yogurt and key lime juice.

**STORAGE TIP:** You can enjoy these dessert cups right away or cover them with plastic wrap and store them in the refrigerator for up to 2 days.

. . . . . . . . . . . . . . . . . . . . . . . . . . . . . . . . . . . . . . . . . . . . . . . . . .

**Per Serving** Calories: 219; Total fat: 13g; Carbohydrates: 18g; Fiber: 0g; Protein: 8g; Calcium: 111mg; Sodium: 63mg; Potassium: 168mg; Vitamin D: 0mcg; Iron: 1mg; Zinc: 1mg

# Pear Trifle

✔ BUDGET-SAVER

✔ VEGETARIAN

**SERVES 2**

**PREP TIME:** 10 MINUTES, PLUS 30 MINUTES TO CHILL

**COOK TIME:** 5 MINUTES

1 (14.5-ounce) can juice-packed sliced pears, drained

¼ teaspoon nutmeg

1 cup 1 percent milk

1 egg yolk

2 tablespoons granulated sugar

2 tablespoons half-and-half

1 tablespoon cornstarch

¼ teaspoon pure vanilla extract

4 fresh mint leaves (optional)

When it comes to managing your food budget and reducing food waste, canned fruit is an excellent choice. Canned pears make this dessert quick and easy to make. This dessert helps to meet your goals with two servings of fruit and a serving of dairy. Be sure to watch the cream mixture closely while cooking it, as it can burn quickly.

1. In a small bowl, mix the pears with the nutmeg and set aside.

2. In a small saucepan, stir together the milk, egg yolk, sugar, and half-and-half over medium heat.

3. Quickly whisk in the cornstarch and stir constantly for 1 minute. Add the vanilla and stir until the mixture begins to bubble, then reduce the heat to low. Continue cooking until the custard is slightly thickened, 4 to 5 minutes more.

4. Remove the saucepan from the heat and chill the custard in the refrigerator for 30 minutes.

5. Spoon some of the custard evenly into the bottom of two small dessert dishes or parfait glasses. Add a quarter of the sliced pears to each portion. Spoon more custard onto the pears and repeat until all of the pears and custard are used.

6. Garnish with fresh mint (if using) and serve.

**VARIATION TIP:** Use a fresh pear and poach the slices in a saucepan of water for 10 minutes or until very tender.

. . . . . . . . . . . . . . . . . . . . . . . . . . . . . . . . . . . . . . . . . . . . . . . . . . . . . . . .

**Per Serving** Calories: 203; Total fat: 4g; Carbohydrates: 37g; Fiber: 3g; Protein: 6g; Calcium: 185mg; Sodium: 76mg; Potassium: 315mg; Vitamin D: 2mcg; Iron: 1mg; Zinc: 1mg

# Fruit Stuffed Baked Apples

✔ ONE-POT
✔ VEGAN

**SERVES 2**

**PREP TIME:** 15 MINUTES
**COOK TIME:** 45 MINUTES

¼ cup brown sugar

¼ cup finely chopped
  dried apricots

3 tablespoons
  chopped walnuts

1 teaspoon avocado oil

½ teaspoon
  ground cinnamon

¼ teaspoon ground nutmeg

2 Gala apples, cored

Fruit provides a terrific base for a healthy DASH dessert. These apples stuffed with a sweet and crunchy filling satisfy your sweet tooth while providing vitamins and healthy fats. If you're feeling indulgent, serve these pretty baked apples warm with a small scoop of vanilla ice cream or frozen yogurt. (Use non-dairy ice cream to keep the dish vegan.)

1. Heat the oven to 375°F.

2. In a small bowl, stir together the sugar, apricots, walnuts, oil, cinnamon, and nutmeg until combined.

3. Slice a thin piece off the top of each apple, creating a flat top. Peel the top one-third of each apple. Place the apples into a small baking dish. Divide the filling between the apples, stuffing it into their cavities and creating a mound on the top of each one. Add a half-inch of water to the baking dish.

4. Bake the apples for 40 to 45 minutes, or until they are soft, and serve.

**SUBSTITUTION TIP:** You can use any baking apple (such as honeycrisp, Braeburn, or Granny Smith). You could also substitute 3 tablespoons of nutty granola for the walnuts.

. . . . . . . . . . . . . . . . . . . . . . . . . . . . . . . . . . . . . . . . . . .

**Per Serving** Calories: 338; Total fat: 10g; Carbohydrates: 64g; Fiber: 7g; Protein: 3g; Calcium: 61mg; Sodium: 11mg; Potassium: 475mg; Vitamin D: 0mcg; Iron: 1mg; Zinc: 1mg

# Mini Greek Yogurt Fruit Tarts

**MAKES 4 TARTS**

**PREP TIME:** 15 MINUTES

**For the Crust**

2 sheets graham crackers

½ cup walnuts,
 finely chopped

2 teaspoons brown sugar

1 teaspoon avocado oil

½ teaspoon cinnamon

Nonstick cooking spray

**For the Filling**

1 cup plain, nonfat
 Greek yogurt

2 teaspoons honey

¼ teaspoon almond extract

4 large strawberries, sliced

½ cup blueberries

4 fresh mint
 leaves (optional)

Canned whipped
 cream (optional)

Dessert is supposed to be a decadent indulgence at the end of a meal, but when you're living a DASH lifestyle it's an efficient way to add more fruit to your diet. Consuming three to four servings of fruit a day is important on DASH because it helps ensure that you get adequate amounts of potassium and antioxidants. These tarts are a twist on a parfait, nestled in a golden homemade tart crust. They can be put together ahead of time and frozen, then defrosted, as long as you wait to add the fresh fruit until the frozen tarts have thawed.

## To Make the Crust

1. Place the graham crackers between two pieces of wax paper and crush them with a rolling pin. Transfer the crumbs to a small bowl. Add the walnuts, sugar, oil, and cinnamon and stir to combine.

2. Spray 4 (4-ounce) ramekins with cooking spray. Divide the crumbs between the ramekins, pressing them into the bottoms and sides of the cups to form the tart crusts.

## To Make the Filling

3. In a small bowl, stir together the yogurt, honey, and almond extract. Evenly divide the mixture between the ramekins.

4. Top each with the berries and garnish with mint leaves and whipped cream (if using). Serve.

**VARIATION TIP:** You can use flavored nonfat Greek yogurt in place of plain, but omit the honey.

. . . . . . . . . . . . . . . . . . . . . . . . . . . . . . . . . . . . . . . . . . . . . .

**Per Serving (1 tart)** Calories: 211; Total fat: 12g; Carbohydrates: 21g; Fiber: 2g; Protein: 6g; Calcium: 114mg; Sodium: 76mg; Potassium: 268mg; Vitamin D: 0mcg; Iron: 1mg; Zinc: 1mg

# Black Bean Brownies

**MAKES 9 BROWNIES**

**PREP TIME:** 15 MINUTES

**COOK TIME:** 30 MINUTES

Nonstick cooking spray

1 (14-ounce) can
 low-sodium black beans,
 rinsed and drained

⅔ cup brown sugar

½ cup dark cocoa powder

2 large eggs

3 tablespoons canola oil

½ teaspoon baking powder

½ cup semisweet chocolate
 chips, divided

2 tablespoons toffee bits

These moist and rich chocolaty brownies are decadent enough that you would never guess they conceal a hefty portion of healthy black beans. High in potassium, B vitamins, magnesium, iron, and fiber, black beans give this dessert such a boost that you may not even consider it dessert! The bits of rich toffee and scattering of chocolate chips elevate this dessert to an addictive level.

1. Preheat the oven to 350°F. Spray an 8-by-8-inch baking pan with cooking spray.

2. Put the beans, sugar, cocoa powder, eggs, oil, baking powder, and 6 tablespoons of the chocolate chips in a food processor. Process until smooth.

3. Pour the batter into the prepared pan. Sprinkle the remaining chocolate chips and the toffee bits over the top of the batter.

4. Bake the brownies for 30 minutes.

5. Remove from the oven and allow to cool. Cut into 9 brownies and serve.

**STORAGE TIP:** Store the brownies in an airtight container at room temperature for 3 days or in the freezer for up to a month.

. . . . . . . . . . . . . . . . . . . . . . . . . . . . . . . . . . . . . . . . . . . . . . . . . .

**Per Serving (1 brownie)** Calories: 214; Total fat: 9g; Carbohydrates: 32g; Fiber: 5g; Protein: 5g; Calcium: 48mg; Sodium: 23mg; Potassium: 322mg; Vitamin D: 0mcg; Iron: 2mg; Zinc: 1mg

# Chewy Oatmeal Cookies

**MAKES 12 COOKIES**

**PREP TIME:** 15 MINUTES
**COOK TIME:** 10 MINUTES

½ cup whole-wheat flour

¼ teaspoon baking powder

¼ teaspoon cinnamon

1 overripe banana

¼ cup peanut butter

2 tablespoons brown sugar

2 tablespoons avocado oil

¼ cup rolled oats

1 large egg

½ teaspoon vanilla

¼ cup walnuts, chopped

It's always terrific to have recipes that use overripe bananas because they seem to ripen in the car on the way home from the store. These healthy cookies fit the bill. Adding a potassium-rich banana to the other ingredients helps reduce the need for both sugar and added fats. The nuts and avocado oil used in place of standard butter also replace saturated fat with healthy fats.

1. Heat the oven to 350°F. Line a baking sheet with parchment paper or a silicone mat.

2. In a medium bowl, stir together the flour, baking powder, and cinnamon and set aside.

3. Mash the banana in a medium bowl. Add the peanut butter, brown sugar, and oil and mix until smooth. Add the oats, egg, and vanilla. Stir until combined.

4. Add the banana-oat mixture to the dry ingredients and stir until a soft dough forms. Stir in the nuts.

5. Place 2 teaspoons of dough per cookie onto the baking sheet.

6. Bake the cookies for 8 to 10 minutes. Let them cool on the baking sheet for 2 minutes before transferring them to a cooling rack.

**STORAGE TIP:** Store in an airtight container in the refrigerator for 5 days or freeze for up to 3 months.

. . . . . . . . . . . . . . . . . . . . . . . . . . . . . . . . . . . . . . . . . . . . . . .

**Per Serving (1 cookie)** Calories: 122; Total fat: 7g; Carbohydrates: 12g; Fiber: 1g; Protein: 3g; Calcium: 17mg; Sodium: 8mg; Potassium: 115mg; Vitamin D: 0mcg; Iron: 1mg; Zinc: 0mg

# No-Bake Mad DASH Cookies

✓ **30 MINUTES OR LESS**
✓ **ONE-POT**
✓ **VEGETARIAN**

**MAKES 12 COOKIES**

**PREP TIME:** 10 MINUTES

¾ cup granulated sugar

¼ cup low-fat milk

4 tablespoons avocado oil

2½ tablespoons
  baking cocoa

1½ cups rolled oats

¼ cup sunflower seeds

¼ cup walnuts, chopped

Traditional no-bake cookies are loaded with sugar because boiling this sweet ingredient creates a syrup that hardens when cooled, creating the structure for the cookie. These treats do contain sugar, but in a significantly reduced amount that conforms to DASH-friendly guidelines. The cookies still hold together with the limited sugar, which is splendid because they are packed with nutrient-rich seeds and nuts.

1. Line a baking sheet with parchment paper.

2. In a large saucepan, stir together the sugar, milk, oil, and cocoa over medium-low heat until the mixture boils. Reduce the heat to low and cook until the sugar melts, stirring constantly, about 2 minutes.

3. In a small bowl, combine the oats, seeds, and nuts until well mixed. Add the oat mixture to the cocoa mixture and stir until combined.

4. Drop the cookie mixture by the tablespoonful onto the prepared baking sheet. Allow the cookies to cool completely, then gently transfer them to a sealed container.

**VARIATION TIP:** To reduce calories and sugar, you can substitute half a cup of allulose for the same amount of sugar in the recipe.

**STORAGE TIP:** You can enjoy these immediately or refrigerate them for up to a week.

. . . . . . . . . . . . . . . . . . . . . . . . . . . . . . . . . . . . . . . . . . . . . . . . . . . . . . . . . . . .

**Per Serving (1 cookie)** Calories: 203; Total fat: 9g; Carbohydrates: 27g; Fiber: 3g; Protein: 5g; Calcium: 23mg; Sodium: 3mg; Potassium: 149mg; Vitamin D: 0mcg; Iron: 1mg; Zinc: 1mg

# Peanut Rice Crisp Bars

**MAKES 8 BARS**

**PREP TIME:** 15 MINUTES

2 cups crisp rice cereal

¼ cup honey

¼ cup crunchy
  peanut butter

Sometimes you just crave something sweet. Desserts, by nature, are not nutritious, but you can modify a recipe to make it a bit better. Remember those crispy rice treats from your childhood? These are a slightly healthier version. The rice cereal provides vitamins $B_6$, $B_{12}$, and D as well as riboflavin, thiamin, folic acid, and iron. Instead of sugary marshmallows, the glue in these treats is honey and peanut butter. Remember, sweets are fine if portioned properly and enjoyed as an occasional treat.

1. Line a 9-by-5-inch loaf pan with parchment paper.

2. Put the cereal in a medium bowl.

3. Put the honey and peanut butter in a small microwave-safe bowl. Heat for 30 seconds in the microwave on high. Remove and stir the mixture, then microwave it for 30 more seconds at 50 percent power.

4. Pour the honey mixture over the cereal and stir to combine.

5. Transfer the cereal mixture to the loaf pan, pressing it into the bottom.

6. Set the pan aside at room temperature to cool. When the mixture has cooled, cut it into 8 equal bars.

**STORAGE TIP:** Store the bars in an airtight container at room temperature for up to a week.

. . . . . . . . . . . . . . . . . . . . . . . . . . . . . . . . . . . . . . . . . . . .

**Per Serving (1 bar)** Calories: 94; Total fat: 4g; Carbohydrates: 14g; Fiber: 1g; Protein: 2g; Calcium: 4mg; Sodium: 2mg; Potassium: 70mg; Vitamin D: 0mcg; Iron: 1mg; Zinc: 0mg

# Pumpkin Custard

✔ MAKE-AHEAD
✔ ONE-POT
✔ VEGETARIAN

**SERVES 4**

**PREP TIME:** 10 MINUTES
**COOK TIME:** 35 MINUTES

Nonstick cooking spray

1 cup canned
  pumpkin purée

½ cup milk

1 large egg

2 tablespoons maple syrup

1 teaspoon ground pumpkin
  pie spice

¼ teaspoon canola or
  avocado oil

2 tablespoons chopped
  pecans or walnuts

Are you a pumpkin pie enthusiast? If so, this scrumptious little dessert will suit you well. You will not overindulge because this treat is perfectly portioned into ramekins and sans crust. Pumpkin is loaded with beta carotene and potassium, so this dessert can even serve as a half portion of vegetables on your DASH plan. Also, you get part of a dairy serving out of it, as well.

1. Preheat the oven to 350°F. Spray 4 (4-ounce) ramekins with cooking spray.

2. In a medium bowl, mix the pumpkin, milk, and egg until blended. Add the syrup and pumpkin pie spice and mix until combined.

3. Heat the oil in a small skillet over medium heat and add the nuts. Toast the nuts for 1 to 2 minutes, stirring constantly. Remove the nuts from the heat.

4. Evenly divide the pumpkin mixture between the ramekins. Top with the toasted nuts. Place the ramekins in a 9-by-11-inch baking dish.

5. Add half an inch of water to the dish and bake for 25 to 30 minutes, until firm.

6. Remove the custards from the oven, allow them to cool slightly at room temperature, and serve them warm.

**INGREDIENT TIP:** Be sure to use plain puréed pumpkin, not pie filling.

**STORAGE TIP:** Store covered with plastic wrap in the refrigerator for up to 5 days.

. . . . . . . . . . . . . . . . . . . . . . . . . . . . . . . . . . . . . . . . . . . . . .

**Per Serving** Calories: 112; Total fat: 5g; Carbohydrates: 14g; Fiber: 2g; Protein: 4g; Calcium: 74mg; Sodium: 35mg; Potassium: 224mg; Vitamin D: 0mcg; Iron: 1mg; Zinc: 1mg

# Banana Cocoa Drop Cookies

✔ **30 MINUTES OR LESS**
✔ **MAKE-AHEAD**
✔ **ONE-POT**
✔ **VEGETARIAN**

**MAKES 12 COOKIES**

**PREP TIME:** 10 MINUTES
**COOK TIME:** 15 MINUTES

2 overripe bananas
½ cup rolled oats
¼ cup cocoa powder
2 tablespoons honey
½ cup peanut butter

Cookies don't need to be complicated to be spectacular; the five simple ingredients in this recipe combine into a drop cookie bursting with banana and peanut butter flavor. You can whip these up in a jiffy because the ingredients (other than the bananas) are probably in your pantry right now. Eat these cookies as an energy-packed mid-afternoon snack on the go.

1. Preheat the oven to 350°F. Line a baking sheet with parchment paper.

2. In a small bowl, mash the bananas. Using an electric hand mixer or a whisk, beat in the oats, cocoa powder, and honey. Beat in the peanut butter until well combined.

3. Drop 12 heaping tablespoons of batter onto the baking sheet and bake for 15 minutes.

4. Cool for 10 minutes before serving.

**STORAGE TIP:** Store in an airtight container at room temperature for 5 days.

. . . . . . . . . . . . . . . . . . . . . . . . . . . . . . . . . . . . . . . . . . . . . . . . . . .

**Per Serving (1 cookie)** Calories: 122; Total fat: 6g; Carbohydrates: 15g; Fiber: 2g; Protein: 4g; Calcium: 12mg; Sodium: 3mg; Potassium: 205mg; Vitamin D: 0mcg; Iron: 1mg; Zinc: 1mg

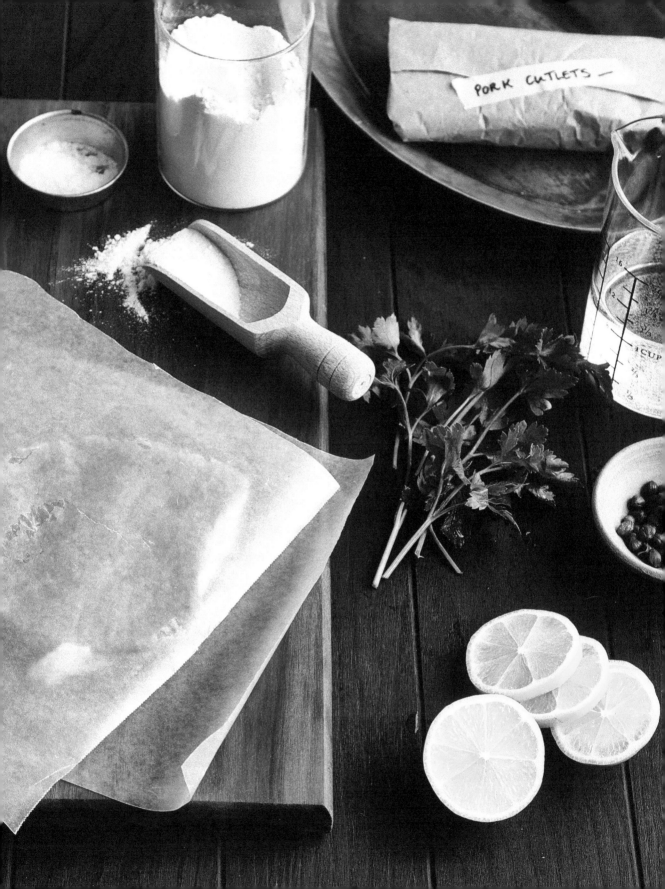

# Measurement Conversions

| | US STANDARD | US STANDARD (OUNCES) | METRIC (APPROXIMATE) |
|---|---|---|---|
| **VOLUME EQUIVALENTS (LIQUID)** | 2 TABLESPOONS | 1 FL. OZ. | 30 ML |
| | ¼ CUP | 2 FL. OZ. | 60 ML |
| | ½ CUP | 4 FL. OZ. | 120 ML |
| | 1 CUP | 8 FL. OZ. | 240 ML |
| | 1½ CUPS | 12 FL. OZ. | 355 ML |
| | 2 CUPS OR 1 PINT | 16 FL. OZ. | 475 ML |
| | 4 CUPS OR 1 QUART | 32 FL. OZ. | 1 L |
| | 1 GALLON | 128 FL. OZ. | 4 L |
| **VOLUME EQUIVALENTS (DRY)** | ⅛ TEASPOON | | 0.5 ML |
| | ¼ TEASPOON | | 1 ML |
| | ½ TEASPOON | | 2 ML |
| | ¾ TEASPOON | | 4 ML |
| | 1 TEASPOON | | 5 ML |
| | 1 TABLESPOON | | 15 ML |
| | ¼ CUP | | 59 ML |
| | ⅓ CUP | | 79 ML |
| | ½ CUP | | 118 ML |
| | ⅔ CUP | | 156 ML |
| | ¾ CUP | | 177 ML |
| | 1 CUP | | 235 ML |
| | 2 CUPS OR 1 PINT | | 475 ML |
| | 3 CUPS | | 700 ML |
| | 4 CUPS OR 1 QUART | | 1 L |
| | ½ GALLON | | 2 L |
| | 1 GALLON | | 4 L |
| **WEIGHT EQUIVALENTS** | ½ OUNCE | | 15 G |
| | 1 OUNCE | | 30 G |
| | 2 OUNCES | | 60 G |
| | 4 OUNCES | | 115 G |
| | 8 OUNCES | | 225 G |
| | 12 OUNCES | | 340 G |
| | 16 OUNCES OR 1 POUND | | 455 G |

| | FAHRENHEIT (F) | CELSIUS (C) (APPROXIMATE) |
|---|---|---|
| **OVEN TEMPERATURES** | 250°F | 120°C |
| | 300°F | 150°C |
| | 325°F | 180°C |
| | 375°F | 190°C |
| | 400°F | 200°C |
| | 425°F | 220°C |
| | 450°F | 230°C |

# References

Appel, Lawrence J., Frank M. Sacks, Vincent J. Carey, et al. November 16, 2005. Journal of the American Medical Association. Effects of protein, monounsaturated fat, and carbohydrate intake on blood pressure and serum lipids: results of the OmniHeart randomized trial. DOI: 10.1001/jama.294.19.2455.

Appel, Lawrence J., M.D., M.P.H.; Thomas J. Moore, M.D.; Eva Obarzanek, Ph.D., et al. April 17, 1997. *New England Journal of Medicine*. A Clinical Trial of the Effects of Dietary Patterns on Blood Pressure. DOI: 10.1056/NEJM199704173361601.

Bergeron, Nathalie, Sally Chiu, Paul T. Williams, et al. February 2016, American Journal of Clinical Nutrition Comparison of the DASH (Dietary Approaches to Stop Hypertension) diet and a higher-fat DASH diet on blood pressure and lipids and lipoproteins: a randomized controlled trial DOI: 10.3945/ajcn.115.123281.

Blumenthal, James A., Ph.D.; Michael A Babyak, Ph.D.; Alan Hinderliter, M.D., et al. January 25, 2010. *Archives of Internal Medicine*. Effects of the DASH diet alone and in combination with exercise and weight loss on blood pressure and cardiovascular biomarkers in men and women with high blood pressure: the ENCORE study. DOI: 10.1001/archinternmed.2009.470.

Center for Disease Control. Hypertension Prevalence and Control Among Adults: United States, 2015–2016. Accessed February 3, 2020. cdc.gov/nchs/products/databriefs/db289.htm.

Comparison of the DASH (Dietary Approaches to Stop Hypertension) diet and a higher-fat DASH diet on blood pressure and lipids and lipoproteins: a randomized controlled trial, American Journal of Clinical Nutrition. academic.oup.com/ajcn/article/103/2/341/4564756.

Environmental Protection Agency. Reducing Wasted Food at Home. Accessed on February 5, 2020. epa.gov/recycle/reducing-wasted-food-home.

Harsha, D. W., F. M. Sacks, E. Obarzanek, et al. February 2004. Hypertension, Effect of dietary sodium intake on blood lipids: results from the DASH-sodium trial. DOI: 10.1161/01.HYP.0000113046.83819.a2.

Harvard Health Publishing. OmniHeart Diets Provide More Options for Heart Health. Accessed on February 4, 2020. health.harvard.edu/PDFs/OmniDiets.pdf.

National Institutes of Health. Vitamin K. Accessed February 4, 2020. ods.od.nih.gov /factsheets/vitaminK-HealthProfessional.

Steinberg, Dori, Ph.D., M.S., R.D.; Gary G. Bennett, Ph.D.; and Laura Svetkey, M.D. April 18, 2018. *Journal of the American Medical Association*. The DASH Diet, 20 Years Later. DOI: 10.1001/jama.2017.1628.

U.S. News Best Diets: How We Rated 35 Eating Plans. Accessed February 3, 2020. health.usnews.com/wellness/food/articles/how-us-news-ranks-best-diets.

van Ballegooijen, Adriana J., Aivaras Cepelis, Marjolein Visser, et al. April 10, 2017. Hypertension. Joint Association of Low Vitamin D and Vitamin K Status With Blood Pressure and Hypertension. DOI: 10.1160 116.08869.

Wengreen, Heidi, Ronald G. Munger, Adele Cutler, et al. September 18, 2013. *American Journal of Clinical Nutrition*. Prospective study of Dietary Approaches to Stop Hypertension–and Mediterranean-style dietary patterns and age-related cognitive change: The Cache County Study on Memory, Health and Aging. academic.oup.com/ajcn/article /98/5/1263/4577302.

Williamson, Jeff D., M.D., M.H.S.; Nicholas M. Pajewski, Ph.D.; Alexander P. Auchus, M.D., et al. January 28, 2019. *Journal of the American Medical Association*. Effect of Intensive vs Standard Blood Pressure Control on Probable Dementia. DOI:10.1001.

Zade, Mohsen Razavi, Mohammad Hosein Telkabadi, Fereshteh Bahman, et al. April 2016. The effects of DASH diet on weight loss and metabolic status in adults with non-alcoholic fatty liver disease: a randomized clinical trial. DOI: 10.1111/liv.12990.

# Index

# Acknowledgments

I'd like to thank Callisto Media, Anna Pulley, and the entire editing team for making this process seamless.

# About the Author

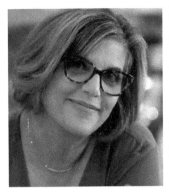

**Rosanne Rust** is an internationally recognized nutrition expert and author with a passion for facts. A researcher and writer at heart, Rosanne created her blog, Chew the Facts (ChewTheFacts.com), to help consumers decipher nutrition fact from myth, so they can relax and enjoy eating for better health. She crafts expert food and nutrition messages that turn confusion into clarity and mistrust into confidence. The owner of Rust Nutrition Services (RustNutrition.com), she also provides nutrition communication services to the food industry and science-based medical organizations.

Rosanne has co-authored several books in the For Dummies consumer series, including *DASH Diet For Dummies, The Glycemic Index Cookbook For Dummies,* and *The Calorie Counter Journal For Dummies.* A wife and mother of three sons, she practices what she preaches: A well-balanced life, which includes food and beverage splurges and an active lifestyle of jogging, walking, weight lifting, yoga, bike riding, golf, kayaking, hiking, boating, skiing, reading, traveling, and of course, good food shared with family and friends.

Follow her on social media @rustnutrition or @chewthefacts.

CPSIA information can be obtained
at www.ICGtesting.com
Printed in the USA
BVHW061741181120
593428BV00004B/4

9 781647 393113